DEDICATIONS

To Rose, Joel, Ari and Talya
for your unending support
and constant inspiration.

To my great teachers, colleagues and students who have always questioned and continue to enlighten my mind "that we may all strive for excellence in the compassionate care of our patients."

Original
Medical Illustrations
by
Virginia Roethemeyer, RNC, CNOR
Fertility Center of North Texas
Dallas, Texas

TABLE OF CONTENTS

MANAGEMENT OF INFERTILITY

A Clinician's Manual

by

BRIAN M. COHEN, M.B.Ch.B., M.D.

Clinical Professor
Dept. of Obstetrics and Gynecology
University of Texas Southwestern
Medical Center at Dallas
Dallas, Texas

2nd Edition

*Essential Medical
Information Systems, Inc.*
Durant, Oklahoma

Direct Mail Orders

Essential Medical
Information Systems, Inc.
P.O. Box 1607
Durant, OK 74702-1607

Telephone Orders

1-800-225-0694

FAX Your Order: (405) 924-9414

SECOND EDITION

ISBN: 0-929240-33-2

Published in the United States 1991

Printed in the United States of America

TABLES

FIGURES

FOREWORD

Dr. Brian Cohen has contributed 13 chapters in various texts, but this is the first book conceived and written solely by the author. I am delighted with his new manual for the management of infertility. This is a straightforward, concise manual which enables the obstetrician/gynecologist to manage successfully the infertile couple and point out the way to parenthood. The text includes chapters in anatomy, physiology of conception, overview of fertility evaluation, diagnostic tests, common problems, current trends (including operative endoscopy), sperm enhancement techniques, GIFT and IVF, and finally basic protocols and therapeutic agents.

In this exciting, fast-changing field of reproduction, it is often difficult to keep up with all that is new and what innovations have stood the test of time. Hopefully newer techniques will emerge, especially in the management of the male. I predict that my friend Brian will keep this meaningful and current text updated with future editions.

ABOUT THE AUTHOR

I have known Dr. Brian Cohen since 1977, shortly after he emigrated from South Africa. He has had superb training in the field of obstetrics and gynecology in Capetown, RSA, Rhodesia, as well as in London at St. Thomas Hospital. He was brought to the USA by the University of Tennessee and became Associate Professor and head of the section of Reproductive Surgery, Division of Reproductive Endocrinology from 1977 through 1980. From 1980 to 1983, he was head of Reproductive Surgery, the Mt. Sinai Medical Center, Cleveland, Ohio. It was here and at Case Western Reserve University where he received his formal fellowship training to become a Diplomat of the American Board of Obstetrics and Gynecology subspecialty of Reproductive Endocrinology. He is presently Clinical Professor at the University of Texas Health Science Center and Director of the Fertility Center of North Texas, Dallas, Texas.

He is known worldwide for his invaluable contributions in the field of reproductive surgery. He is an eminent teacher and has been responsible for numerous "hands on" courses in microsurgery. He has produced three films, including *Vascularized Transplantation of the Fallopian Tube* which was judged "most outstanding film" at the American College of Obstetrics and Gynecology annual film award in 1978.

Melvin R. Cohen, M.D.
Professor Emeritus,
Northwestern University Medical School,
Department of Obstetrics and Gynecology;
Consultant, Division of Reproductive
Endocrinology and Infertility.

#1 Hypothalamic-Pituitary-Gonadal Function in the Male

Anatomy and Physiology

The synchronized functions of the cerebrum, hypothalamus, and pituitary affect the release of gonadotropins (follicle-stimulating hormone [FSH] and luteinizing hormone [LH]), with subsequent hormonal and spermatogenic responses in the testicles (Figure 1.1). FSH plays a primary role in the initiation of spermatogenesis and the function of Sertoli cells, which nourish the developing germ cells in their evolution from spermatocytes and spermatids to mature spermatozoa. Inhibin from the Sertoli's cells plays a role in the negative loop regulation of FSH production.

LH plays a primary role in stimulating interstitial Leydig's cells to produce testosterone. In turn, testosterone elevation suppresses LH secretion.

FSH and LH regulation of the testicles thereby ensures normal maturation of spermatozoa and their adequate nutrition and activation prior to ejaculation.

Sperm production occurs within the testicles. These organs are external so that they may maintain the low temperatures (lower than normal body temperatures) necessary for normal sperm production.

The development and maturation of spermatozoa require approximately 75 days. The first emission of male ejaculate contains most of the spermatozoa. This and subsequent emissions are constituted by secretions of the prostate, seminal vesicles and urethral glands; fluids that facilitate the emission of spermatozoa at the time of orgasm.

Clinical Correlations

Adequate and normal rhythmic function of the hypothalamic-pituitary-gonadal axis ensures LH and FSH stimulation of the testicles for normal sperm production.

Defects of gonadotropin output can be related to:

- Cerebral trauma
- Hypophysectomy
- Pituitary adenoma

Singularly or together, these may contribute to hypogonadotropic hypogonadism with low plasma testosterone and failure of spermatogenesis.

The loss of testicular testosterone and/or inhibin production alternatively can result from damage to the testicles by:

- Previous inflammation
- Toxicity
- Radiation
- Surgical excision

Testicular inhibin and testosterone usually suppress FSH and LH, so that their loss with elevation of gonadotropins is indicative of testicular failure.

Figure 1.1 ➡

FIGURE 1.1 – **Reproductive Physiology of the Male – The Relationship Between Gonadotropins and Sperm Production**

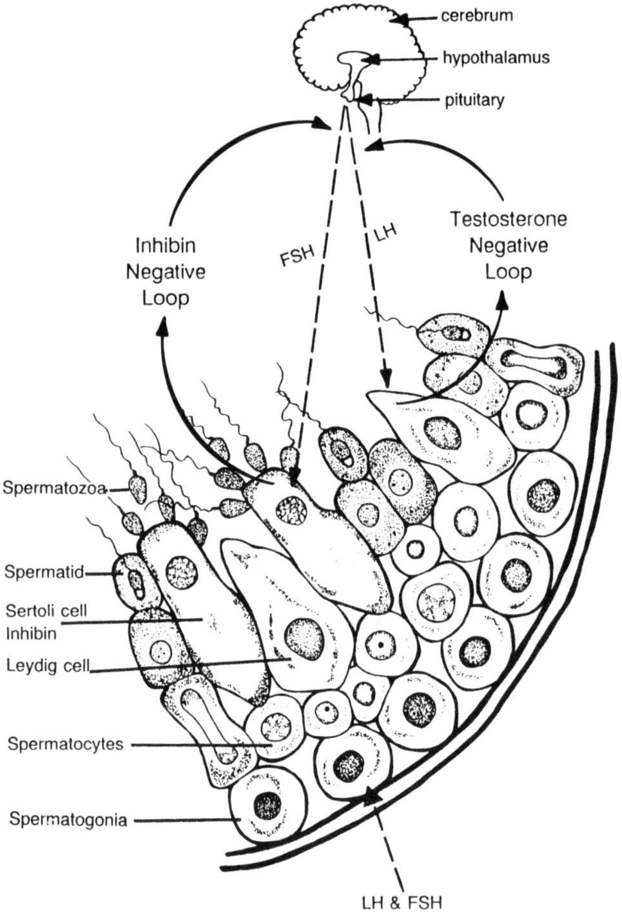

NOTES

#2 Hypothalamic-Pituitary-Gonadal Function in the Female

Anatomy and Physiology

Cerebral cortical activity results from multiple stimuli as a response to the surrounding environment. Cerebral cortical function affects hypothalamic-pituitary-gonadal activity. Multiple cortical stimuli modulate hypothalamic function and the release of gonadotropin-releasing hormone (GnRH), which, in turn, modulates the pituitary release of FSH and LH. The synchronized function of FSH and LH is modulated by ovarian responses, particularly the output of estrogens and progesterone.

Hypothalamic-pituitary function may be altered by:

- Abnormal levels of pituitary prolactin
- Thyroid dysfunction
- Elevated plasma androgens

The general pattern of pituitary and ovarian secretion in a single menstrual cycle is illustrated in Figure 3.1.

Cyclical Ovarian Function

Responding to pituitary gonadotropins, follicles are recruited and stimulated to maturation, with timely production of estrogen and release of a mature ovum at ovulation.

Under FSH stimulation, the dominant follicle is selected from a cohort of follicles in the ovaries during the first four to six days of the cycle. Estradiol is produced by granulosa cells. FSH and estradiol stimulate and induce further FSH and estrogen receptors in these cells. There is a subsequent cascade of estrogen production, which initiates the pre-ovulatory LH surge.

Within the ovary, the dominant follicle suppresses further growth and development of other follicles in its cohort. As estrogen and FSH levels are activated, they, in turn, result in the development of LH receptors in the granulosa and theca cells of the ovary. These produce progesterone during the postovulatory phase of the menstrual cycle.

The first half of the menstrual cycle is dominated by the production of estradiol. At mid-cycle, the LH surge is responsible for:

- Final maturation of the ovum
- Second meiotic division
- Activation of collagenase enzymes
- Rupture of the ovarian surface

This facilitates ovulation and activates the corpus luteum to secrete progesterone, which dominates the hormonal milieu of the second half of the menstrual cycle.

#3 Menstrual Cycle: Response of Female Genital Tract

3. This description is confined to events immediately before ovulation and during the luteal phase of the menstrual cycle (Figure 3.1).

The effects on the female genital tract of the estradiol surge include:

- Cervical – Physicochemical structure of the mucus is penetrable and receptive to spermatozoa. Secretions are maximal in:
  - Amount
  - Clarity
  - Spinnbarkeit
  - Ferning
- Tubal cornu and isthmus – These are relatively closed, facilitating an "egg locking" effect
- Fimbria – These are highly vascularized and erectile, facilitating fimbrial activity close to the surface of the ovary. Fimbrial gonadal approximation is accomplished by vascular engorgement and contractile activity of the:
  - Fimbria ovarica
  - Mesosalpingeal muscles
  - Muscles of the ovarian surface
  - Muscles of the utero-ovarian ligaments
- Ovum pickup – This is facilitated by drawing the fimbria over the surface of the ovary. The fimbrial cilia are highly active, and the sticky cumulus oophorus surrounding the ovum on the surface of the ovary is easily grasped by the cilia, which transport the ovum into the ampulla
- Gametes – These are moved toward the uterus, from the distal to the proximal oviduct, by coordination of:
  - Tubal secretions
  - Cilial activity
  - Muscular contractions
  - Fluid currents

FIGURE 3.1 – **Reproductive Physiology of the Female – The Relationship Between Gonadotropins and Ovarian, Endometrial, Thermal and Cervical Response of the Menstrual Cycle**

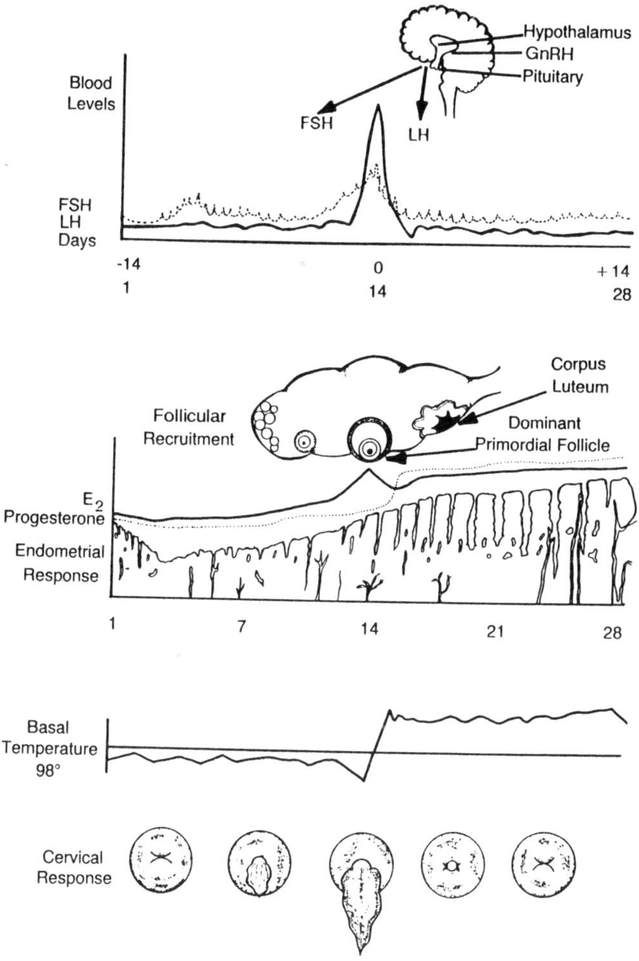

#4 Sperm Cycle in Female

Millions of sperm are deposited in the vagina at intercourse. The initial emission is primarily spermatozoa, and additional secretions propelling the sperm into the vagina are derived from the:

- Seminal vesicles
- Prostate gland
- Urethra

These secretions are rich in alkaline phosphatase and fructose, to facilitate sperm activation and survival in hostile, acidic, vaginal secretions.

The cervical mucus in its most fertile, clear, active, and physicochemical form assists in the selection of healthy, potent, penetrable spermatozoa which proceed rapidly through the female genital tract. Sperm transport is assisted by vaginal contractions during sexual activity. The spermatozoa swim through the relatively obstructed cornu and isthmus, a further process contributing to sperm selection. Thousands of sperm pass through the uterus; hundreds progress through the oviducts and may enter the peritoneal cavity.

The spermatozoa swim actively against the fluid currents and cilial beating patterns of the oviduct, which are synchronized to direct the ovum towards the uterus. This passage through the female genital tract is associated with the phenomenon of "capacitation." Capacitation is currently termed the "acrosome reaction," whereby the acrosome cap on the surface of the spermatozoa head is altered with the release of enzymes which assist in sperm penetration of the zona pellucida. The sperm culminate this final state of activation in the tubal ampulla, where they await ovum capture by the fimbria.

NOTES

#5 Ovulation, Fertilization and Postovulatory Events

5.

Ovulation

Ovulation, triggered by an adequate LH surge, most commonly occurs during days 12 through 14 of a regular 28-day menstrual cycle. The effects of the LH surge are:

- Final maturation of the oocyte
- Induction of the second meiotic division
- Stimulation of collagenase enzymes at the ovarian surface
- Facilitation of ovum release with rupture of the follicular wall, where the cumulus remains adherent to the ovarian surface

The tubal ostium is drawn down to the ovarian surface by the fimbria ovarica. This fimbrial ovarian activity achieves ovum pickup by the fimbrial cilia, which transport the ovum into the tube (Figure 5.1).

Fertilization

Fertilization most commonly occurs in the distal oviduct. As the first spermatozoa penetrates the zona, its acrosome reaction induces a granular response that blocks further sperms from entering the egg, thus preventing polyspermic fertilization.

With the release of the second polar body:

- The second meiotic division is completed
- The sperm and ovum DNA and chromosomes are combined
- Reduction division occurs

Mitosis then continues, with divisions through two-, four-, and eight-cell stages, and the cleaving embryo forms a morula within the zona.

The morula develops into a blastocyst, which is kept within the oviduct until a change in the endocrine status, related to LH surge and progesterone production, occurs. The rise in progesterone and relative change in the estradiol:progesterone ratio alters oviduct dynamics, after which the embryo is transferred into the endometrial cavity.

Postovulatory Effects

The Endometrium

During the menstrual cycle, there is an initial phase of endometrial proliferation; after ovulation, the endometrium enters a secretory phase.

The first half of the cycle is dominated by estrogen, with glandular proliferation and buildup in endometrial receptors. The endometrium is prepared for progesterone activity with adequate secretory function and receptivity to embryonal implantation.

During the postovulatory "secretory" phase of the menstrual cycle, glandular secretory function is optimal. Vascularization of the endometrium increases, with the endometrium becoming thick, velvety and well-defined into spongiosa, compacta and basal layers. Subsequently, further engorgement with decidualization and stromal edema occurs. Immediately prior to menstruation, a perivascular fibroblast reaction occurs, resulting, respectively, in:

- Stromal leukocyte infiltration
- Vascular spasm
- Tissue breakdown
- Menstruation

Details regarding the development, maturation and dating of the endometrium are classically reviewed according to the criteria of Noyes, Hertig, and Rock (Figure 5.2).

The Corpus Luteum

The function of the corpus luteum in the ovary is dependent on its original morphological and functional preparation during the follicular/proliferative phase of the menstrual cycle.

Adequate hormonal stimulation of the follicle will ensure the development of adequate granular and thecal cells. Adequate FSH stimulation results in a buildup of FSH and E_2 receptors, which ensure and facilitate the subsequent buildup of adequate LH receptors.

This adequate cellular and receptor preparation also ensures adequate secretion of progesterone during the second half of the cycle. At the endometrial level, adequate progesterone function is dependent on the adequacy of previous estrogen stimulation and buildup of estrogen and progesterone receptors (progesterone works on previously estrogenized tissue receptor sites [Figure 5.3]).

Progesterone-Dominant Luteal Phase

The postovulatory phase of the menstrual cycle is also known as the progesterone-dominant luteal or secretory phase. If pregnancy is to result, it is during this phase that the following occur:

- Fertilization
- Cleavage
- Tubal transport
- Implantation

Effects on the female genital tract at this point in the cycle include:

- Cervical mucus which:
  - Is dry
  - Is cellular
  - Has a thickened physicochemical structure impermeable to spermatozoa
- Loss of ferning and spinnbarkeit
- Changes of the cornu and isthmus of the oviduct in:
  - Secretory and cilial rhythms
  - Relative relaxation
  - Loss of "egg locking" effect

  The synchronized, timely transfer of the morula to the endometrial cavity occurs at this point
- Oviduct fimbriae and ampulla which:
  - Are less congested
  - Have lost their erectile activity
  - Change in vascular and lymphatic flow patterns
  - Decrease in fluid volume

- Decrease in ciliated cellular activity, with a dominance of secretory cells
- Are active; muscular contractions and rhythms conduct the embryo into the endometrial cavity

- Implantation of morula/blastocyst, which is dependent on:
  - Endometrial receptivity
  - Hormonal interplay between the embryo and endometrium
  - Trophoblastic proliferation and subsequent vascularization
  - HCG secretion by syncytiotrophoblast, picked up in the maternal host approximately 10 days postovulation
  - Maintenance of progesterone output and steroid function of the corpus luteum until replaced by placental function (at the eighth to 10th week of pregnancy)

Figures 5.1, 5.2 and 5.3 ➡

NOTES

FIGURE 5.1 – **Tubo-Ovarian Approximation and Ovum Pickup at Ovulation**

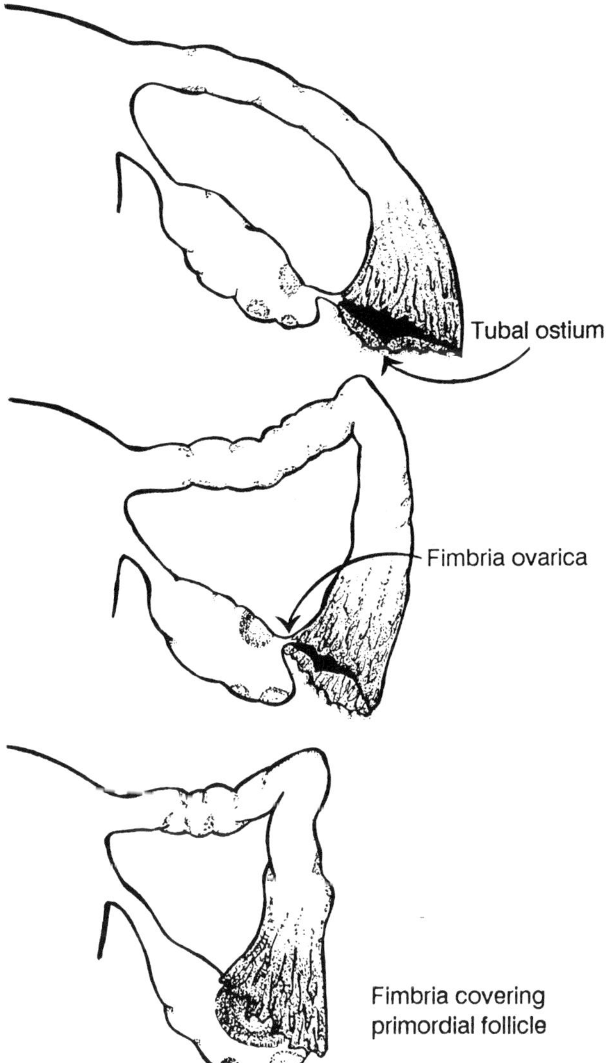

FIGURE 5.2—**Histologic Dating of Endometrium as Described By Noyes, Hertig and Rock (Used for diagnosis and management of luteal phase defect.)**

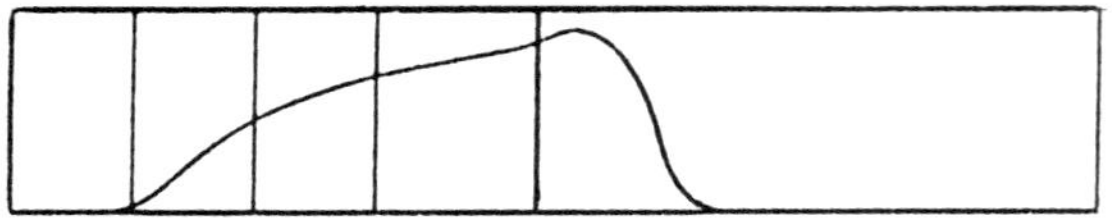

GLAND MITOSES—Gland mitoses indicate proliferation. They occur during menstruation because repair and breakdown are progressing simultaneously at that time.

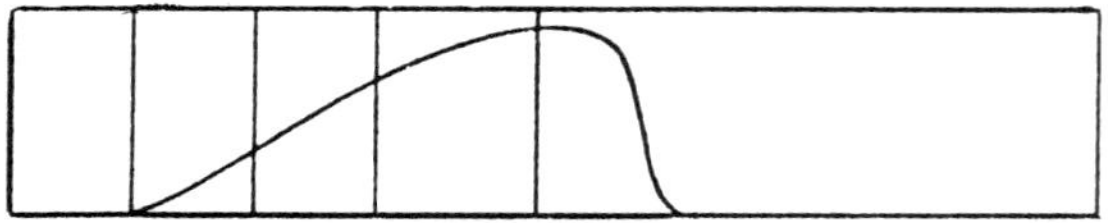

PSEUDOSTRATIFICATION OF NUCLEI—This is characteristic of the proliferative phase but persists until active secretion begins. It is not resumed until the glands have involuted during menstruation.

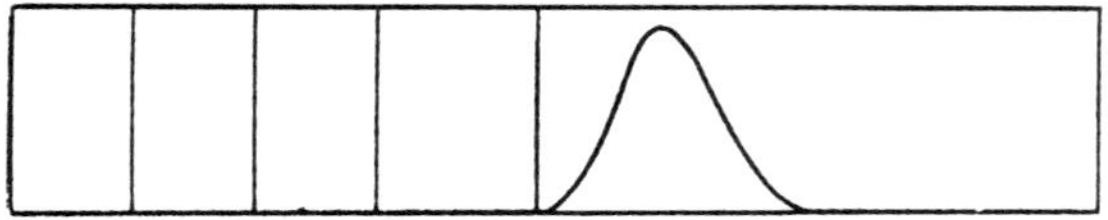

BASAL VACUOLATION—This is the earliest morphological evidence of ovulation found in the endometrium. It begins approximately 36 to 48 hours following ovulation.

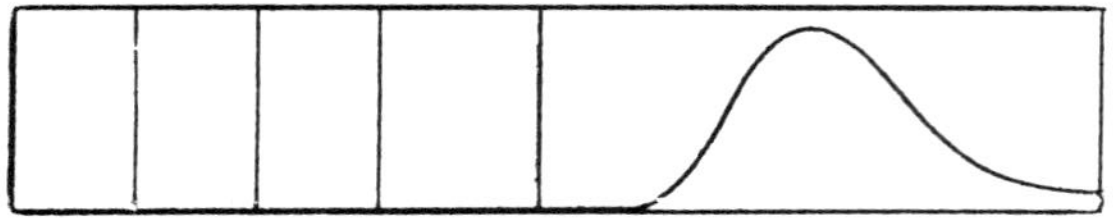

SECRETION—This curve represents visible secretion in the gland lumen, active secretion falls off more abruptly. In the later stages the secretion becomes inspissated.

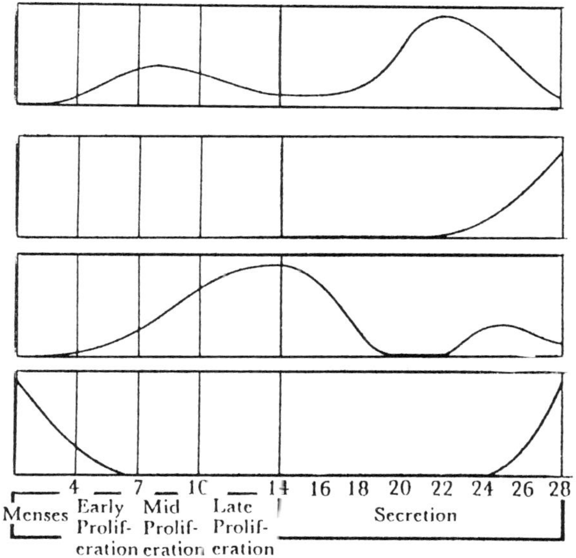

STROMAL EDEMA—This factor varies with the individual, particularly the rise during proliferation which may be almost absent. The edema which accompanies secretion is more constant.

PSEUDODECIDUAL REACTION—This is evident first around the arterioles and progresses until just before menstruation a superficial compact layer is formed.

STROMAL MITOSES—These are most abundant during the proliferative phase, absent during active secretion but reappear during the stage of predecidual formation.

LEUCOCYTIC INFILTRATION—Throughout the cycle there are always a few lymphocyctes. Polymorphonuclear infiltration begins about two days before the onset of flow.

Criteria for histologic dating of the endometrium showing approximate relationship of useful morphologic factors. (Noyes RW, Hertig AT, Rock J: Dating the endometrial biopsy. Fertil Steril 1950;1:3. Reproduced with the permission of the publisher, The American Fertility Society.)

FIGURE 5.3 — **Functional Anatomy – Ovulation to Implantation**

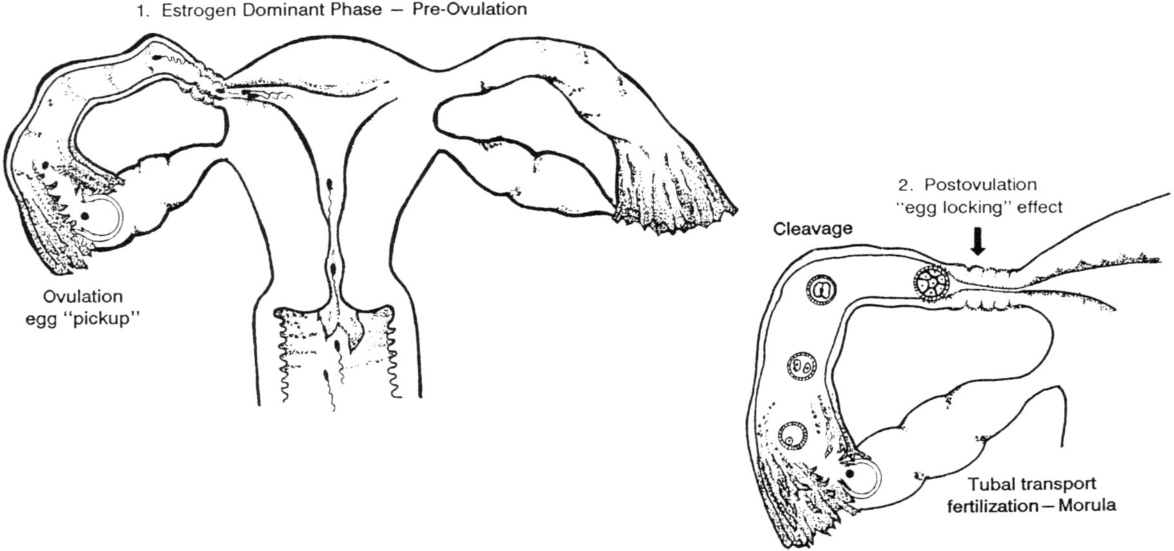

3. Progesterone Dominant Phase – Postovulation
Relaxation of isthmus cornu with
embryo transfer to endometrial cavity.

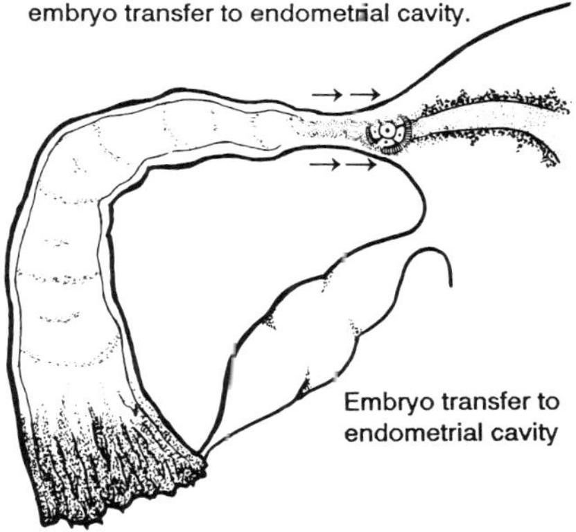

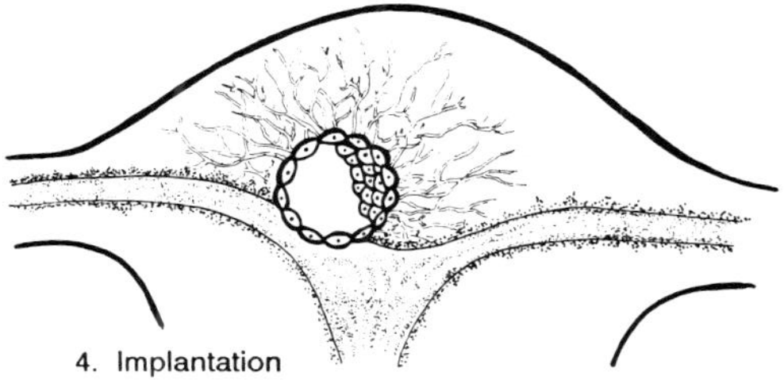

4. Implantation

#6 Clinicopathological Factors

Hormonal Dysfunction Preventing Conception

Hormonal dysfunction, due to disturbance of endocrine rhythms, may prevent conception at many levels. In the hypothalamic-pituitary-ovarian axis, breakdowns may occur at any of the following levels:

- Cerebral
- Hypothalamic
- Pituitary
- Ovarian function

6.

These disturbances may generally result from:

- Stress
- Nutritional disorders, including:
  - Obesity
  - Anorexia
  - Bulimia

Locally, these disturbances may occur as hypothalamic or pituitary lesions, including:

- Traumatic
- Inflammatory
- Neoplastic
  - Adenomas
  - Carcinomas

Normal menstrual function may also be disturbed by dysfunction of other endocrine organs, including the:

- Thyroid
  - Hyperthyroidism
  - Hypothyroidism
- Adrenal
  - Hyperandrogenism
  - Hypercortisolism
- Ovary
  - Hyperandrogenism

Androgens and progestogens act as antiestrogens, meaning that pathological secretion or iatrogenic administration of androgens or progestins may cause multiple endocrine disturbances and resultant ovulatory dysfunction.

Principles of Attaining Conception

Conception is dependent on the synchronized, normal functions of the hypothalamic-pituitary-gonadal axis and the male and female genital organs. Conception occurs when:

- Healthy, normal sperm are deposited in the vagina in a timely manner
- Receptive cervical mucus is present
- An ovum is released at the ovarian surface
- The released ovum is picked up from the ovarian surface
- Hormonal rhythms are timely, preparing an adequate follicle and healthy corpus luteum
- The morula is transferred into the endometrial cavity at the appropriate time
- Luteal function and preparation of the endometrium to facilitate implantation and consequent nourishment of the early embryo is adequate
- Adequate response of the corpus luteum to HCG stimulation results in a continued output of estrogen and progesterone, facilitating the onset of gestation

Couples having intercourse more frequently have a greater chance of achieving conception (Figure 6.1). Sixty percent of normal couples achieve conception within approximately six months. However, age is a contributing factor that causes this percentage to significantly decline after age 35 (Figure 6.2).

Counseling regarding the necessity of patience in those couples undergoing treatment for infertility is of paramount importance. These couples must allow sufficient time for their treatment plan to be effective if they are to accomplish their goal of pregnancy (Figure 6.3).

Summary of Causes, Diagnosis and Treatment

Most problems relating to couples' inability to conceive are diagnosed at eight levels:

- Sperm and male factor (See Section #18)
- Cervical factor (See Section #19)
- Ovulatory and hormonal factors (See Section #20)

- Mechanical factor—Uterine (See Section #21)
- Mechanical factor—Tuboperitoneal (See Section #22)
- Endometriosis (See Section #23)
- Immunological factor (See Section #24)
- Idiopathic (See Section #25)

A diagnosis of infertility is based on:

- Detailed patient history
- Physical examination:
  - General—Multiple endocrine parameters
  - Regional—Lower abdominal examination
  - Local—Pelvic examination
- Simple laboratory tests
  - Blood
  - Urine
- Review of temperature graphs (see Section #9)
- LH surge guide records

Specialized examinations for determining infertility include:

- Pelvic ultrasound
- Hysterosalpingogram
- Endometrial biopsy
- Minor surgical procedures, including:
  - Hysteroscopy
  - Laparoscopy
  - Chromotubation
  - Intraperitoneal biopsy
- Immunological studies of the:
  - Blood
  - Semen
  - Cervical mucus

Causes of infertility are usually multifactorial. Treatment goals are to:

- Remove the cause
- Combat the effects
- Correct anatomical defects
- Supplement and/or correct physiological dysfunctions

The result of treatment, it is hoped, will be the attainment of a healthy, viable conception and live-born child.

Principles of Physician Management

At the initial visit, the physician will:

- Review basic principles of human anatomy and the physiology of conception with the couple
- Review all previous records and investigations, including x-ray films and details of operative reports such as:
  - Diagrams
  - Photo documentation
  - Videos
- Detail complete histories and physical examinations for both partners
- Summarize data
- Define and list the major causes of infertility
- Propose and plan therapy by:
  - Reviewing options
  - Defining time intervals necessary for each option
  - Adequately counseling couples considering a course of therapy
  - Planning specific details, booking procedures and preparing cycles

Figures 6.1, 6.2 and 6.3 ➡

FIGURE 6.1 — **Incidence of Pregnancy Correlated With Frequency of Intercourse**

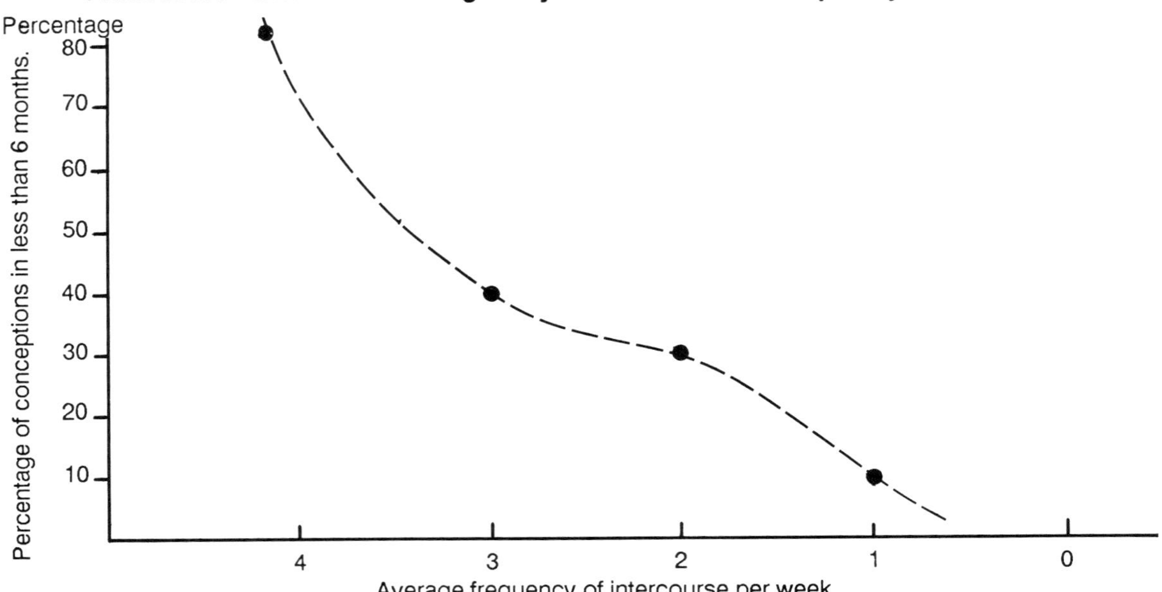

(Modified from Behrman and Kistner, "Progress In Infertility" [1975].)

FIGURE 6.2—**Correlation Between Age and Incidence of Pregnancy Within Six Months**

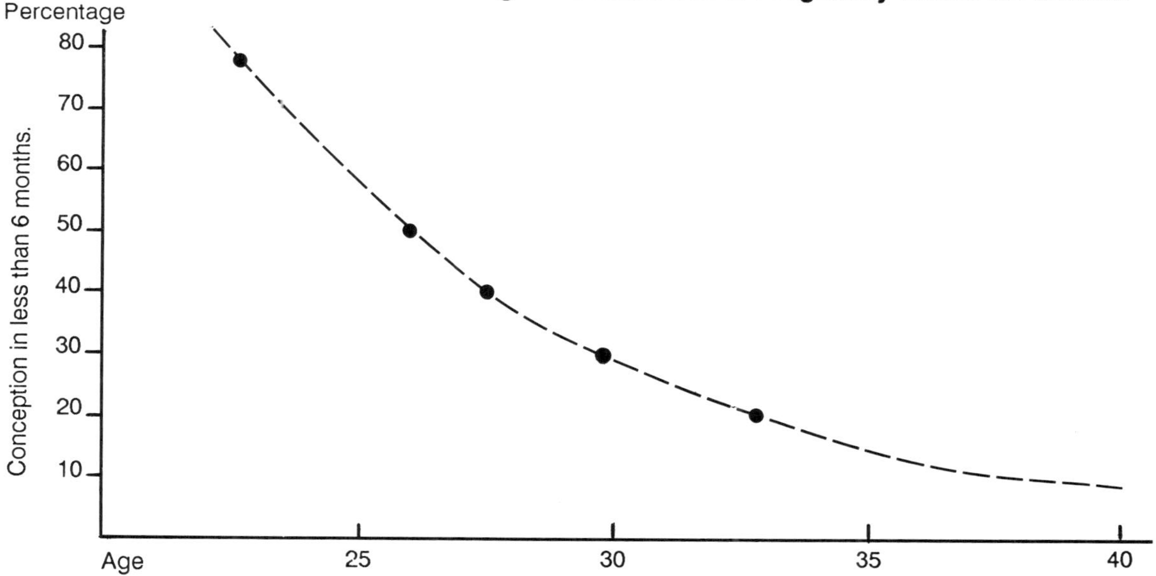

Note that the most significant decline of incidence of pregnancy within six months is at 35 years of age.
(Modified from Behrman and Kistner, "Progress In Infertility" [1975].)

FIGURE 6.3—**Cumulative Incidence of Pregnancy in Young Couples Attempting Conception and Having Regular Intercourse**

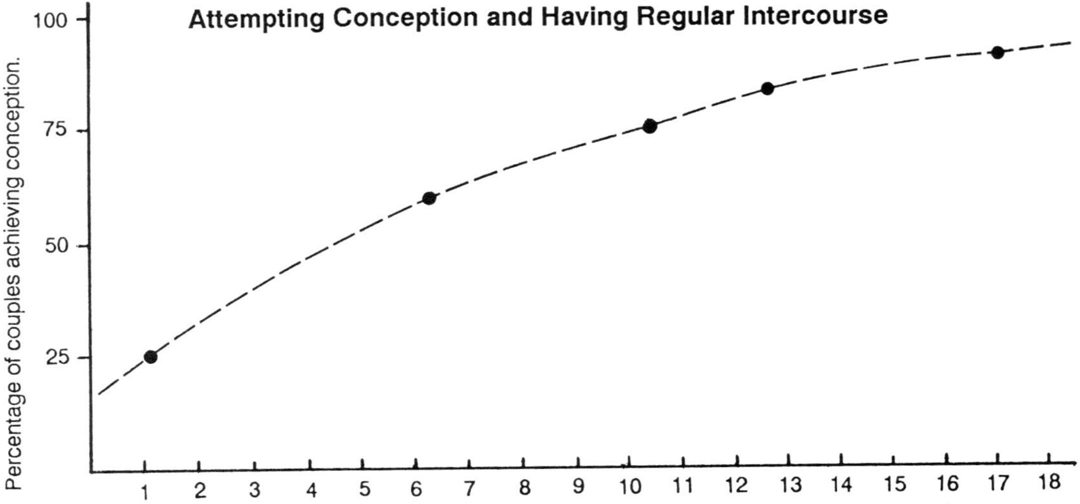

Number of months required for conception. (Time of exposure without conception. **NOTE**: 60% of these couples will have conceived within approximately six months.)

(Modified from Behrman and Kistner, "Progress In Infertility" [1975].)

NOTES

#7 Primary Consultation: History and Physical

The patient history and physical examination, performed during the primary consultation, is directed at assessing the possible causes of infertility relative to the eight levels of factors to be considered (see Section #6).

MALE

History and Physical

7. Factors to be noted in the patient history include:

- Operations on gonads during childhood
- History of mumps
- Testicular trauma
- Inguinoscrotal operations
- History of penile:
  - Discharge
  - Prostatitis
  - Epididymitis

  Culture and/or antibiotic therapy may be indicated if these factors are involved
- History of local or general malignancy–May indicate prior chemotherapy
- Exposure to:
  - Toxins
  - Drugs
  - Cannabis
  - Alcohol
- Heat exposure, eg, hot tubs and saunas
- Tight and/or ill-fitting underwear
- History of hepatitis or chronic liver disease
- History of sexually transmitted diseases (STDs), such as gonorrhea or chlamydia

The physical examination should:

- Exclude varicocele
- Check gonadal size and consistency
- Note normal appearance of urethral meatus (hypospadias)
- Include:
  - Semen analysis (culture sensitivity)
  - Hormonal studies
  - Urological consultation

FEMALE

History and Physical

Factors to be noted in the patient history and physical examination should include:

- Cervical status
- Ovulatory disorder
- Mechanical disorders, including:
  - Uterine
  - Tuboperitoneal
- Endometriosis

Cervical Factor

Factors to be noted in the patient history include:

- Previous surgery
- Previous:
  - Freezing
  - Laser surgery
  - Cautery
- Dyspareunia
- Postcoital bleeding
- Previous infections, including:
  - Cervicitis
  - Positive cultures for gonorrhea, chlamydia and/or mycoplasma
- Abnormal Pap smears and their treatments
- Congenital anomalies
- Maternal diethylstilbestrol (DES) exposure
- Previous dilatations, including:
  - D & C
  - Childbirth delivery
  - Tears
- Hormonal causes, including:
  - Hypoestrogenism
  - Hyperandrogenism
  - Hyperprolactinemia
- Menstrual irregularity
- Hypomenorrhea or oligomenorrhea
- Previous abnormal postcoital tests (PCTs)

The physical examination should determine the status of the cervix regarding:

- Cockscomb
- Pinhole os

- Lacerations
- Ectropion
- Erosion
- Infected secretions
- Mucus:
  - Dryness
  - Thickness
  - Viscousness
  - Cellularity
- Absence of sperm in PCT
- Sperm in PCT:
  - Immobilized
  - Clumped
  - Asthenic

The cervix is to be assessed at mid-cycle (pre-ovulatory) and PCT. If PCTs are abnormal, treatment is indicated.

Ovulatory Disorders

Factors to be noted in the patient history include:

- Mid-cycle pelvic pain
- Dysmenorrhea
- Breast tenderness
- Fluid retention, eg, premenstrual bloatedness
- Late menarche
- Irregular, painless periods or amenorrhea
- Major weight loss or gain
- Lifestyle and stress factors
- Hirsutism and/or virilization
- Galactorrhea
- Headaches and/or visual disturbances
- Previous cerebral injury/disorders, including:
  - Meningitis
  - Encephalitis
  - Coma
- Previous cranial or pituitary surgery
- Previous hormonal injections, eg, medroxyprogesterone acetate (MPA)
- Previous use of oral contraceptives (OCs)
- Flat temperature graph
  - Early or late thermal shift
  - Variations in thermal shift

- Possible premature menopause, with symptoms of:
  - Amenorrhea
  - Hot flashes
  - Insomnia
  - Irritability

The physical examination for ovulatory disorders should include:

- Stressed facies
- General stature
- Body habitus:
  - Obesity
  - Anorexia
  - Ponderal index
- Skin, including:
  - Vellus hair pattern
  - Dryness
  - Acne
- Cushingoid facies
- Hirsutism
- Temporal baldness
- Vaginal dryness
- Clitoromegaly
- Cervix:
  - Dryness (hypoestrogenic)
  - Abundant, clear, ferning mucus (hyperestrogenic)
- Uterus (normal vs. clinically small in size)
- Ovaries (impalpable vs. palpable, possible polycystic)
- Previous endometrial biopsy
  - Proliferative
  - Secretory
  - Dating of endometrium for possible luteal phase defect
- Plasma progesterone:
  - 4 to 8 ng/mL – Ovulated but inadequate level
  - 9 to 15 ng/mL – Borderline
  - 15 to 25 ng/mL or greater – Normal

- Additional hormonal studies, including:
  - Gonadotropins (FSH and LH)
  - Prolactin
  - Androgens (testosterone, DHEAS and androstenedione)
  - TSH, T_3 and T_4
  - Cortisol
  - E_2 and E_1

Mechanical Disorders—Uterine

Factors to be noted in the patient history should include:

- DES exposure
- Menorrhagia
- Increase or decrease in menstrual flow
- Unilateral or atypical dysmenorrhea
- Previous D & C sepsis (postabortion)
- Termination of pregnancy
- Recurrent miscarriage
- Premature delivery
- Postpartum hemorrhage
- Retained placenta
- Known uterine scarring
- Previous resection of uterine adhesions and/or polyps
- Previous use of intrauterine device (IUD)
- Complicated caesarian section

The physical examination will reveal:

- Impression of small uterus
- Broad uterus
- Fibroids
- Tenderness

Should any of these be revealed with the physical examination, the following additional tests are recommended:

- Hysterosalpingogram
- Hysteroscopy
- Endometrial biopsy

Mechanical Disorders – Tuboperitoneal

Factors to be noted in the patient history include:

- History of pelvic inflammatory disease (PID)
- Drainage of pelvic abscess
- DES exposure
- Previous IUD use with recurrent:
  - Bleeding
  - Infection
- Sexual history (multiple partners, etc.)
- Previous pelvic surgery, including:
  - Ovarian cystectomy
  - Uterine surgery
  - Caesarian section
- Previous appendectomy
- Previous exploratory laparotomy
- Major upper abdominal surgery
- Previous tubal surgery
- Sterilization
- Previous tubal pregnancy
- Previous removal of tube
- Tubal conservation
- Known endometriosis

Factors to be noted in the physical examination include:

- Cervical discharge
- Uterine or adnexal tenderness
- Parametrial or adnexal thickening or palpable masses
- Pelvirectal uterosacral thickening or tender nodularity
- Enlarged palpable ovaries

Additional tests include:

- Complete blood count (CBC) and sedimentation rate
- Cervical culture for:
  - Chlamydia
  - Mycoplasma
  - Ureaplasma

- Sonogram for:
  - Hydrosalpinges
  - Ovarian cysts
  - Venous engorgement
  - Endometriosis
    - Fixed organ sign, eg, ovary to posterior uterus
- Hysterosalpingogram, to exclude spasm
- Hysteroscopy
- Laparoscopy
- Chromotubation
- Biopsy (possibly) of:
  - Peritoneum
  - Ovary

Endometriosis

The patient history regarding overall diathesis should reveal whether or not the individual is:

- Energetic and active
- Compulsive
- Obsessive
- Goal- or career-oriented
- Bright, dynamic
- A high achiever
- Ambitious
- Emotionally high-strung
- Of low body weight with a low percentage of body fat (usual)
- DES exposured
- Intolerant of cold, especially in the hands and feet
- Experiencing no symptoms

If the patient experiences dysmenorrhea, it classically occurs on the first day of menses and may be associated with:

- Nausea
- Diarrhea (frequent bowel and urinary symptoms)
- Feelings of hotness and coldness (retrograde menstruation)

Cyclic aggravation of perimenstrual or periovulatory pain will occur with deep dyspareunia, while superficial dyspareunia may be related to vaginal dryness.

Menstrual abnormalities may include:

- Increased flow
- Shorter cycle (with ovarian endometriomas)
- Pre- or postmenstrual spotting
- Short luteal phase
- Cyclic:
    - Diarrhea, blood staining
    - Recurrent urinary infections (culture negative)
    - Bladder irritation at menstruation

Abdominal and/or pelvic pain may be experienced as:

- General and non-specific
- Mid-cycle accentuation (ovarian activity with possible periovarian adhesions)
- Menstrual aggravation
- Unilateral/bilateral
- Central
- Deep vaginal
- Radiating:
    - To the back (uterosacral)
    - Down the inner thigh (possible ovarian enlargement or fixity)

Factors to be noted in the physical examination include:

- General disposition
- Cold periphery
- Fibroadenosis of breasts
- Abnormal tenderness of abdomen
- Pelvic masses
- Vaginal dryness
- Inappropriate absence of cervical mucus (hypoestrogenic)
- Cervical hemorrhagic "spots"
- Cervical lateral displacement
- Palpable tender areas reproducing sensation of dyspareunia
- Tender paracervical areas
- Tender, possibly enlarged, palpable ovaries
- Tense, possibly nodular, thickened, tender uterosacral ligaments (pelvirectal exam)

- Cul-de-sac tenderness and/or masses
- Rectovaginal nodularity

Additional tests include:

- HSG for determination of:
  - Uterine displacement
  - Convoluted, saccular dilatation, usually with patent oviducts
  - Loculated spill
- Laparoscopy for:
  - Panoramic view
  - Biopsy and systematic assessment of pelvis
  - Detailed assessment of:
    - Peritoneum
    - Ovaries (ovarian fossa when elevated)
    - Cul-de-sac
    - Uterosacral ligaments
    - Tubo-ovarian relationships
- Staging for AFS classification (see Section #16)

Overview: Re-Options of Therapy

Therapeutic options include:

- Medical:
  - Expectant management
  - Supplemented ovulation induction
  - Suppression of:
    - BCP
    - Progestin
    - Danazol (Danocrine®)
    - GnRH agonist
- Surgical:
  - Operative endoscopy
  - Associated laser surgery:
    - CO_2
    - Argon
    - KTP-532
    - Sapphire-tipped YAG

    In selected cases, surgery includes nerve ablation
    - Laparotomy, including selective modified presacral neurectomy

- Combinations of therapeutic options, with pre- and postoperative hormonal suppression

Immunological Factors

The male immunological factors to be noted in the patient history and physical examination include:

- History of recurrent prostatitis
- Testicular injuries
- Previous inguinoscrotal surgery
- Vasectomy
- Abnormal sperm viscosity and clumping
- Asthenospermia
- Azoospermia
- Sperm agglutination (head to head or tail to tail)

The female immunological factors to be noted in the patient history and physical examination include:

- Recurrent abnormal PCT tests showing:
  - Immotile sperm
  - Sluggish movement of sperm
  - Sperm with non-purposeful movement
- Confirming the timing of PCT with normal mucus, assessing:
  - Sperm/mucus interaction
  - Activity with donor sperm/donor mucus (in crossmatch tests [Figure 12.2])

Additional tests include:

- Sperm antibody tests (Kibrick, Franklin, and Dukes)
- Immunobead antibody tests, including:
  - IgA
  - IgM
  - IgG

Idiopathic Infertility

A diagnosis of idiopathic infertility is accomplished by the meticulous exclusion of all other factors through detailed review of the patient history, results of the physical examination and of all other special investigations.

#8 Planning of Investigation and Treatment

The timing of investigations and the procedures of testing in relation to phases of the menstrual cycle are crucial to an accurate diagnosis of the causes of infertility and the treatment of those causes (Figures 3.1 and 8.1).

Non-invasive tests should be performed initially, with additional indicated tests performed on the principle of the least to the most invasive.

The initial visit should include the following routines:

- Institute temperature graph
- Obtain cervical cultures for:
  - Chlamydia
  - Mycoplasma
  - Ureaplasma
  - Pap smear (if indicated)
- Perform hormonal testing (blood work); this should be performed in the morning during the proliferative phase of the cycle and prior to the physical examination
- Document and/or counsel regarding coital problems and sexual frequency
- Refer for psychological counseling if indicated
- Advise couples regarding the timing of tests (Figure 8.1)

8.

Timing of Tests

Tests should be timed as follows:

- Blood work – Drawn during days two to six of the cycle; the tests include levels of:
  - FSH
  - LH
  - Prolactin
  - Testosterone
  - Free testosterone
  - DHEAS
  - 17-hydroxyprogesterone
  - E_1
  - E_2
  - TSH, T_3 and T_4

- Hysterosalpingogram – Performed between cycle days seven and nine
- Postcoital tests and mucus/sperm evaluation – Performed prior to the temperature rise, between cycle days 11 and 13
- Plasma progesterone – Drawn seven days post-temperature rise, usually between cycle days 20 and 22
- Endometrial biopsy – Performed 12 days after the temperature rise and after confirming negative βHCG, usually between cycle days 26 and 28
- Hysteroscopy/laparoscopy – Performed between days eight and 10. Associated operative (laser) laparoscopy may be performed at this time, if indicated (see Section #6)

Figure 8.1 ➜

FIGURE 8.1 — **The Infertility Evaluation — Proposed Timing of Investigations**

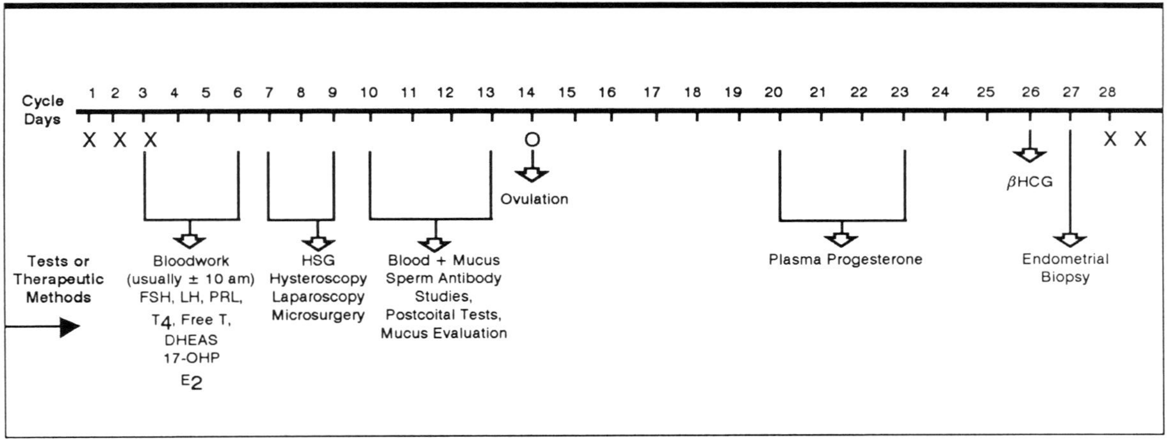

NOTES

#9 The Temperature Graph

The temperature graph is a helpful guide to basic hormonal activity relative to ovulation and the production of progesterone. In principle, progesterone activates thermal centers and causes an elevation of basal body temperature (BBT). The BBT graph, therefore, reflects:

- The onset of progesterone secretion
- Maximal thermal change observed
- The duration of progesterone output

The thermal shift (postovulation) is usually 0.4 to 0.6 degrees F. Review of the temperature graph over a few months provides a simple indication of the cycle length and may suggest repetitive abnormal functions, such as:

- Flattened anovulatory chart
- Recurrent elongated follicular phase
- Recurrent slow, staggered thermal shift
- Recurrent short luteal phase
- Recurrent fluctuations in luteal thermal activity

These and other variations of the expected chart compatible with regular ovulatory menstrual cycles may suggest the need for:

- Generalized hormonal testing
- Measurement of mid-luteal progesterone level
- Evaluation of timed endometrial biopsy

Basic Methodology

The temperature is taken for two to three minutes orally upon awakening and before any physical activity. Temperature results are recorded daily on a suitable graph.

A basal thermometer may simplify the reading of the temperature, since its marked graduations are widespread. Electronic thermometers may also be used.

Large graph paper is preferred since it provides a magnified pattern that facilitates easy evaluation of temperature changes. The temperature graph may be scrutinized to review:

- A simple overview of cycle length
- Follicular/proliferative vs. secretory/luteal phase
- The nature of the thermal shift

Figure 9.1 illustrates the appearance of a temperature graph for a "normal" ovulatory woman. There are usually 14 days on either side of the ovulatory thermal shift (within two days). The mid-cycle rise is adequate if it is greater than 0.6 degrees F and occurs over a 48-hour period. There is a constant elevation with a maintained luteal shift.

Basic diagnostic review patterns suggesting the need for further evaluation include:

- Anovulation (Figure 9.2)
- Ovulatory dysfunction
  - Possible secretory/luteal phase defect (Figure 9.3)
  - Short secretory/luteal phase (Figure 9.4)
- A slow thermal shift, indicating a possible defect in LH surge (Figure 9.5)
- Long follicular/proliferative phase (Figure 9.6)
- Short follicular/proliferative phase with normal secretory/luteal phase (Figure 9.7)
- Short follicular/proliferative phase with short secretory/luteal phase (Figure 9.8)

Overall temperature graph abnormalities indicate the need for a detailed history, physical examination and hormonal testing so that hormonal abnormalities that cause or contribute to these variations can be identified. All causes of anovulation or ovulatory dysfunction include:

- General cerebral-hypothalamic dysfunction
  - Physiological
  - Stress
  - Weight and nutrition problems, including:
    - Obesity
    - Anorexia
    - Bulimia
  - Previous trauma

- Previous inflammation
- Previous tumors
  - Benign
  - Malignant

Also related to general cerebral dysfunction are:

- Hypothalamic-pituitary dysfunction (in addition to pituitary), including:
  - Trauma
  - Inflammation
  - Infarction
  - Tumors (prolactinomas)
- Gonadal, including:
  - Failure and/or premature menopause
  - Ovulatory dysfunctions and anovulation related to hyperandrogenism
    - Polycystic ovarian syndrome
    - Hyperthecosis
- Thyroid:
  - Hypothyroidism
  - Hyperthyroidism
- Adrenal:
  - Hyperandrogenism, including late onset congenital adrenal hyperplasia and enzyme defects
- Iatrogenic:
  - Post medications
  - Depot progestogens
  - Long-term, combination estrogen/progestin pills

Principles of Testing

Causes of ovulatory dysfunction are discussed in Section #20. Testing should include:

- Selective measurement of gonadotropins, including:
  - FSH
  - LH
- Pregnancy testing, ie, βHCG
- TSH, T_3 and T_4 levels
- Progesterone levels from days 21 to 22

- Androstenedione, DHEAS, 17-hydroxyprogesterone
- Testosterone and/or free testosterone
- Timed endometrial biopsy on or after cycle day 26

Treatment

Treatment includes counseling and therapy for:

- Weight gain to attain ideal weight
- Weight loss to lower body fat percentage
- Stress management
- Correction of specific hormonal abnormalities:
  - Bromocriptine for hyperprolactinemia
  - Low-dose dexamethasone for adrenal hyperandrogenism
- Correction of endometriosis, if related to defective ovulation and/or luteal phase defect, by:
  - Medication
  - Surgery

Ovulatory treatment includes:

- Use of clomiphene citrate
- Selective use of:
  - HCG (injection)
  - HMG
  - FSH
- Use of progesterone vaginal suppositories
- Assisted use of GnRH agonists
- Combinations of the above

Close review and detailed assessment of a daily BBT provides clues to the possibility of hormonal/ovulatory dysfunction in many patients. These suggestive patterns should alert suspicion and indicate the need for meticulous exclusion of an endocrine or dysfunctional ovulatory factor as the cause of infertility (see Section #20).

FIGURE 9.1 — **Basic Temperature Graph Appearance in "Normal" Ovulatory Woman**

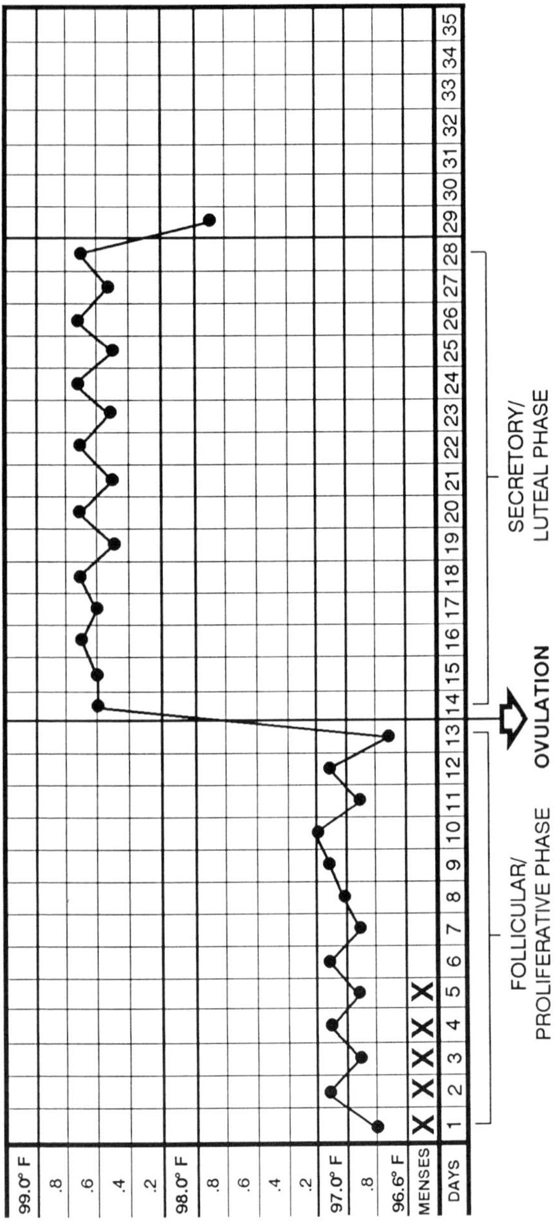

FIGURE 9.2 — **Temperature Graph — Anovulation**

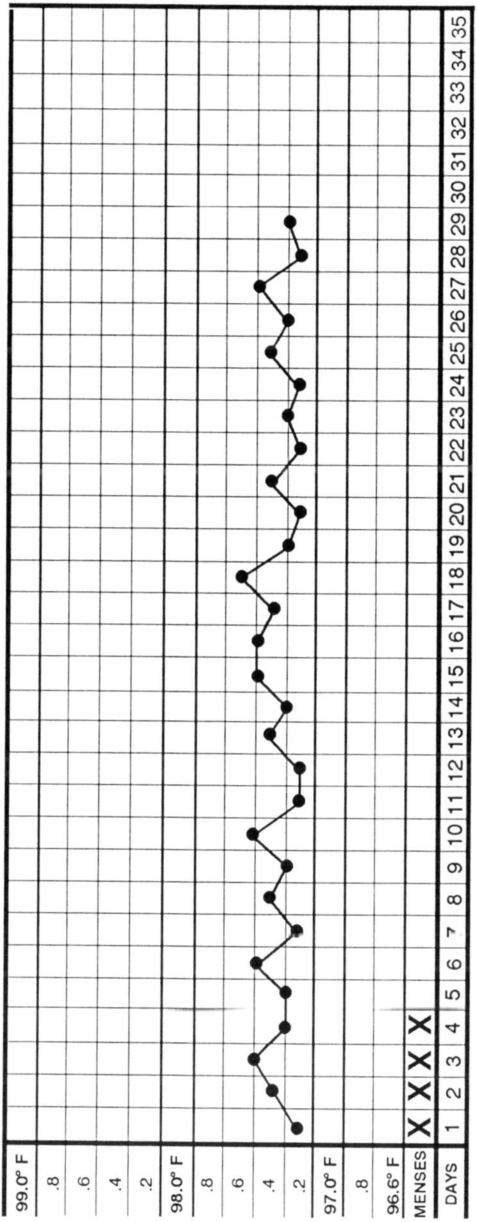

FIGURE 9.3—**Temperature Graph—Ovulatory Dysfunction, Possible Secretory/Luteal Phase Defect**

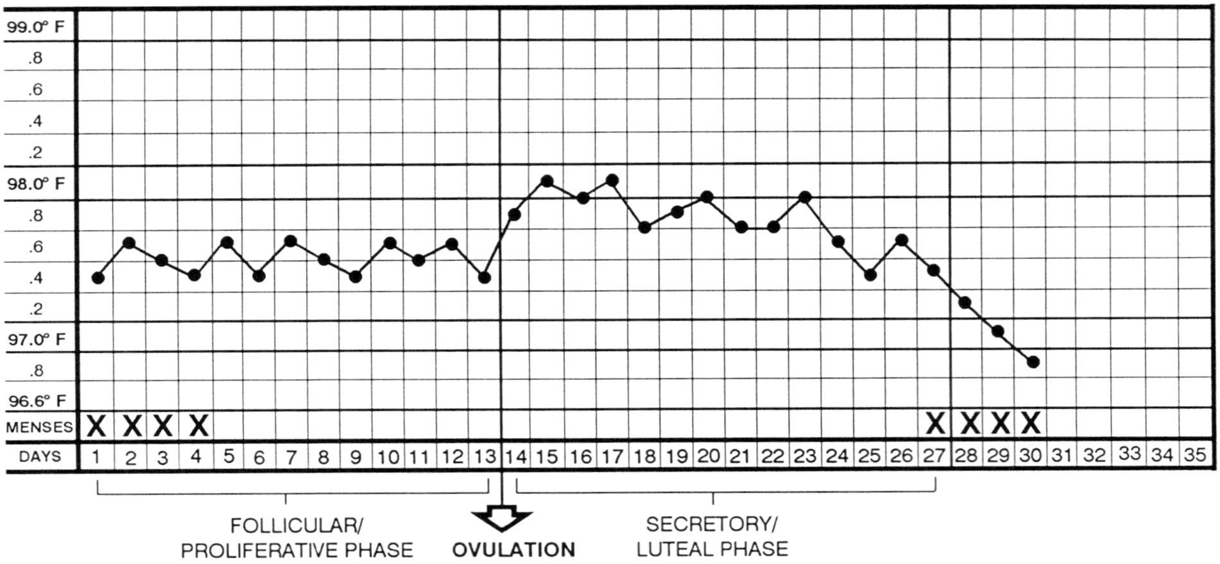

FIGURE 9.4 — **Temperature Graph — Ovulatory Dysfunction, Short Secretory/Luteal Phase**

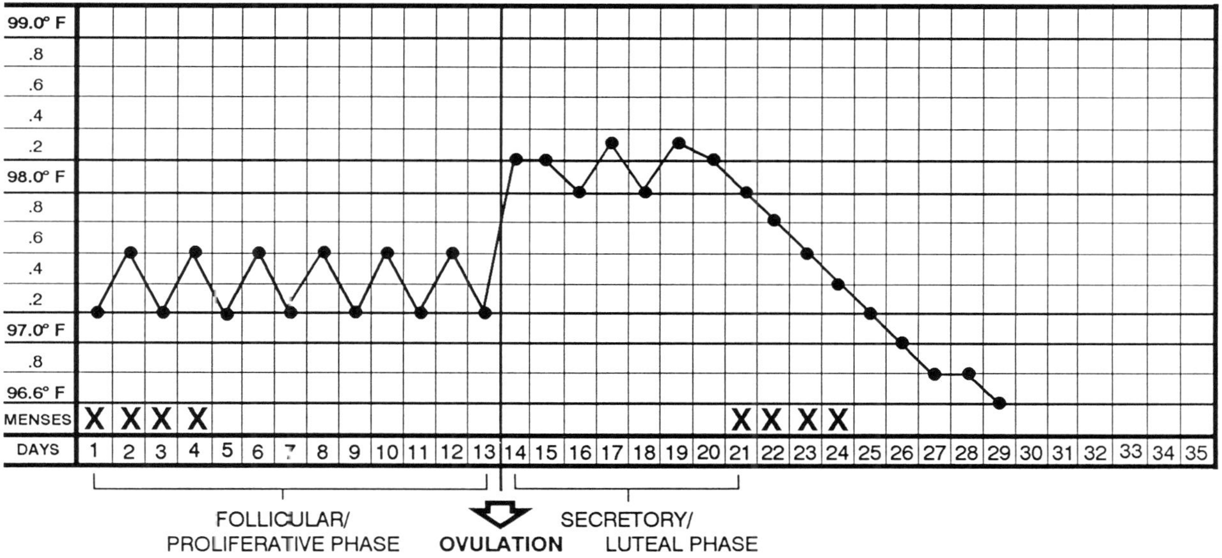

FIGURE 9.5 – **Temperature Graph – Slow Thermal Shift, Possible Defect in LH Surge**

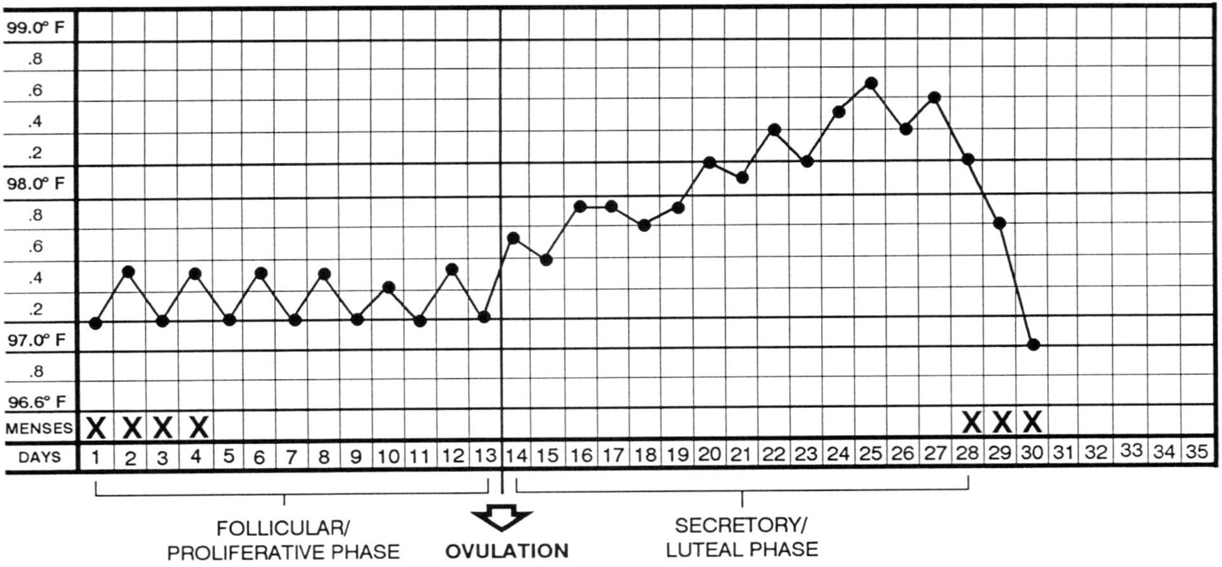

FIGURE 9.6 — Temperature Graph — Long Follicular/Proliferative Phase

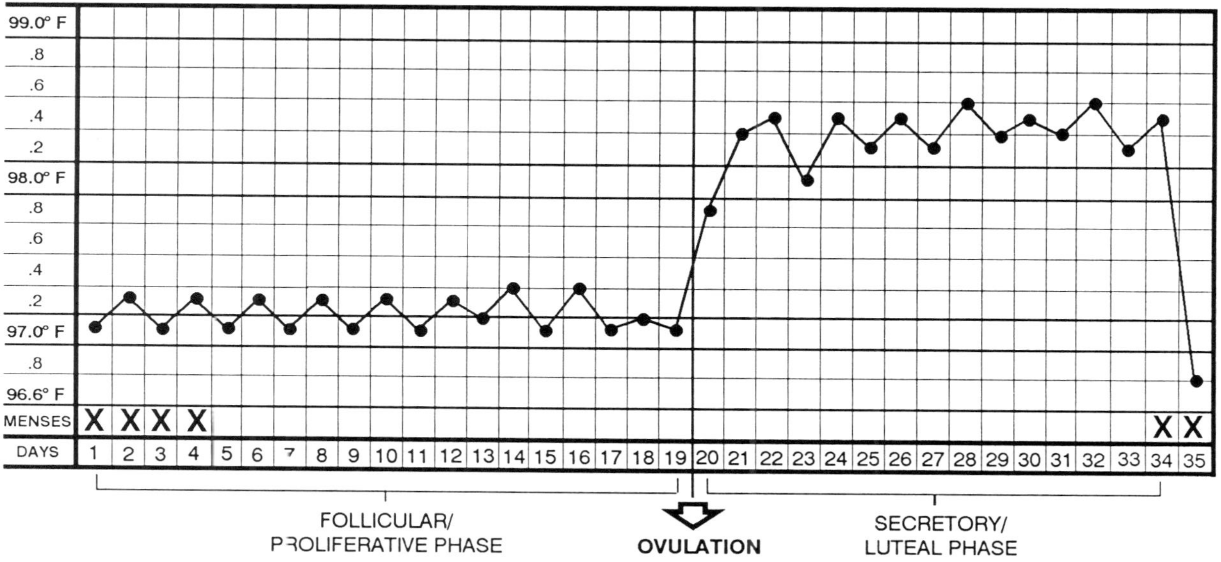

FIGURE 9.7 – **Temperature Graph – Short Follicular/Proliferative Phase, Normal Secretory/Luteal Phase**

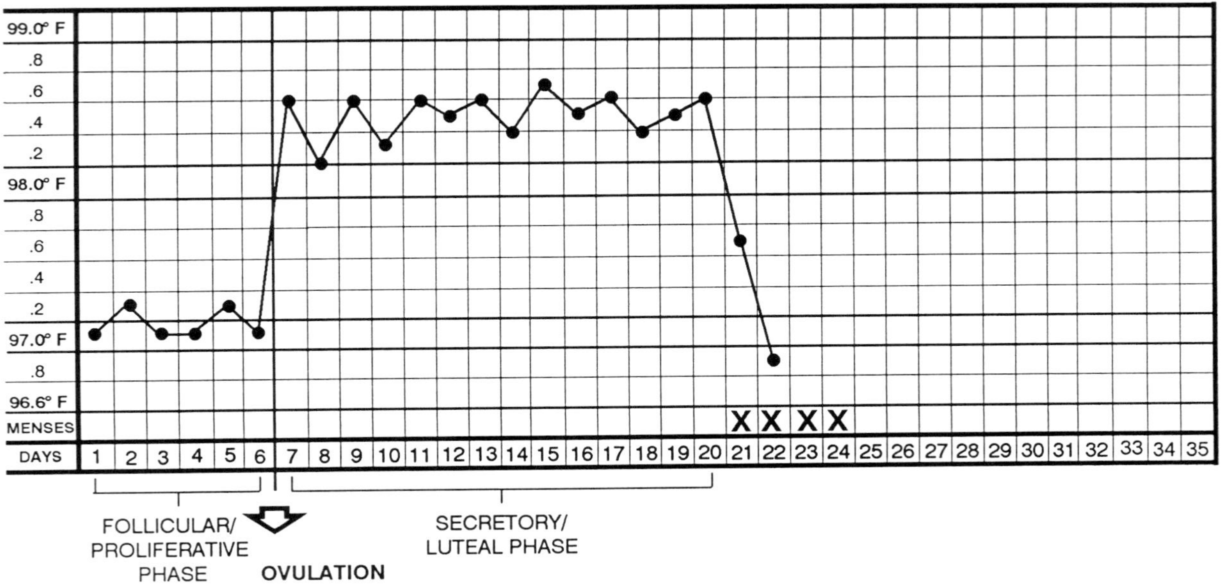

FIGURE 9.8 – **Temperature Graph – Short Follicular/Proliferative Phase, Short Secretory/Luteal Phase**

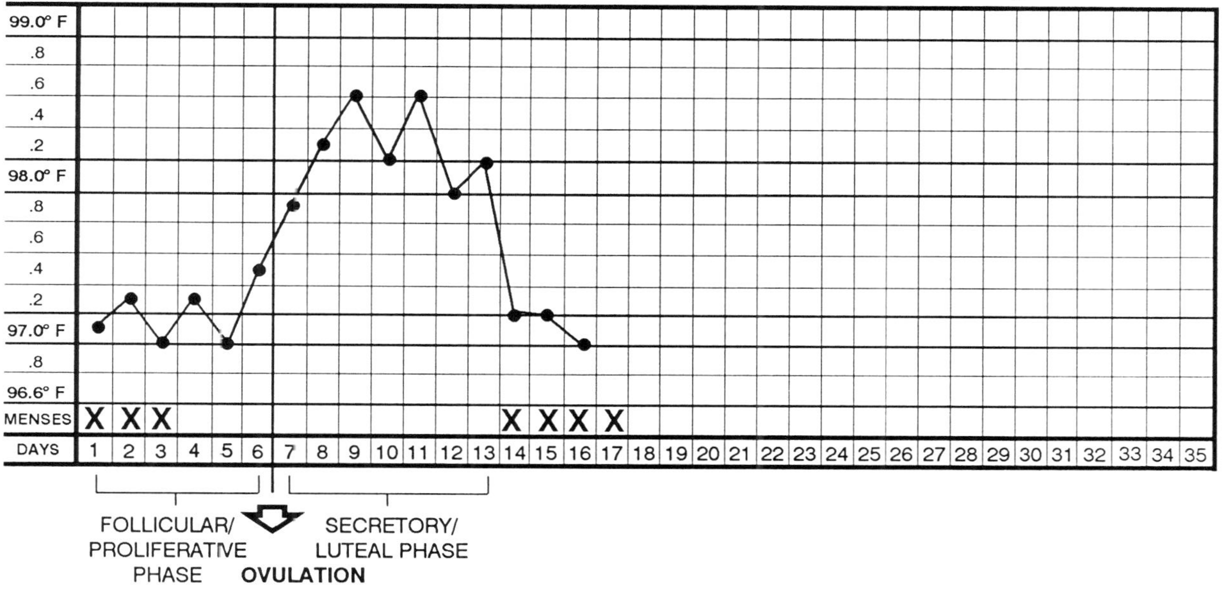

#10 Semen Analysis

Semen Collection/Analysis Factors

Semen analysis is an integral part of the evaluation of infertility. Sperm for such analysis is collected in a sterile jar made of inert material. Collection is by masturbation or partner manipulation following two days of sexual abstinence. Ideally, the sample is obtained at the laboratory, but the specimen may be produced at home if it is delivered to the laboratory within two hours of emission.

The coagulum is allowed to liquify for 20 to 30 minutes and is then examined for the following parameters:

- Volume per mL
- Numbers per mL
- Motility (percentage motile vs. necrospermia)
- Quality of motility (grade non-deviating forward progression vs. asthenospermia)
- Morphology, including percentages of:
  - Normal forms
  - Number of abnormal forms (head, neck, and/or tail defects)
- Presence or absence of:
  - Agglutination (head to head, neck to neck and tail to tail)
  - Leukocytes
  - Fructose
  - Pus cells–Indication of pyospermia
  - Red blood cells–Indication of hematospermia
- Bovine mucus penetration test–mL per hour
- Computerized assessment of quality and numbers with movement showing adequate forward progression and non-deviating head progression
- Nude (zona free) hamster egg penetration test. The minimum percentage of eggs penetrated should be 10 to 14, though the most fertile commonly range from 30 to 80 percent

Factors of a normal specimen include:

- Volumes of one to three mL
- Counts of 40 to 100 million per mL
- Motility of greater than 80 percent
- Morphology of greater than 60 percent normal forms
- Absence of leukocytes
- Presence of fructose
- Early liquefaction and vigorous progressive movement
- Bovine mucus penetration greater than 35 mm per hour

Possible Abnormalities

Hypovolemia

An abnormal specimen showing hypovolemia (ie, volumes less than one mL after two days of sexual abstinence) may result in:

- Inadequate numbers of sperm remaining close to the cervix
- Recurrent negative postcoital tests revealing few or no sperm in the cervical mucus

For couples with hypovolemia, fertility is best achieved by artificial insemination (direct placement of the low volume of sperm into the cervical mucus [see Section #28]).

Hypervolemia

Hypervolemia (ie, volumes greater than five mL) may result in dilution of sperm, particularly when associated with low numbers (eg, 10 million per mL). A five mL sample delivering 50 million sperm, for example, may be diluted to a functional count of only 10 million per cc.

The treatment procedure for hypervolemia involves the collection of split ejaculate. Since most of the sperm is passed at first emission (see Section #1), it is collected separately from the remainder of the ejaculate and then used for artificial insemination (see Section #28).

Sperm Quality

Although sperm counts above 20 million per mL generally indicate fertility, the quality of the sperm is the major determining factor. A sperm sample having a count of 20 million per mL with greater than 80 percent morphologically normal, motile spermatozoa exhibiting non-deviating forward progression offers greater chances of fertility than a sperm sample which consists of a count of 20 million per mL and which is associated with a low percentage of normal forms and/or motility.

Closer scrutiny of the female partner is indicated if oligospermia (sperm counts of less than 20 million per mL) is associated with sperm of excellent quality. In this case, it is probable that a combined factor of a borderline fertile male with an associated abnormality of the female exists.

The laboratory semen analysis must be correlated with a well-timed PCT (see Section #12), since the activity of the sperm *in vivo* is the true standard of its functional capacity.

In view of the current prevalence of sexually transmitted diseases (STDs), all semen samples undergo a routine sperm culture. Symptoms of prostatic or male genital infection indicate the need for prostatic massage and urethral sampling for specialized cultures, such as:

- Chlamydia
- Trichomonas
- Ureaplasma infection
- Mycoplasma infection

Sperm Antibody Testing

See Section #24.

Basic Physiology

See Section #1.

If significant abnormalities of the semen analysis and/or PCT are found, the patient should be referred to an urologist for further evaluation.

Causes of Abnormal Semen Analysis

An abnormal semen analysis may be the result of:

- Previous:
  - Prostatitis
  - Testicular injury
  - Testicular/scrotal surgery
  - Vasectomy (with or without vasovasostomy)
  - Non-descent of testicles and subsequent surgery
- Epididymitis
- Congenital atresia of the duct collecting system
- Alcoholism
- Hepatitis/liver disease
- Drugs/toxins
- Chemotherapy
- Radiation

A basal workup is suggested, including:

- Semen analysis
- Prostatic massage
- Urethral culture for sensitivity, plus:
  - Specific chlamydia
  - Ureaplasma
  - Mycoplasma
- Hormonal testing, including:
  - LH
  - FSH
  - Prolactin
  - TSH, T_3 and T_4
- Vasogram
- Special tests, including:
  - Mucus penetration
  - Hamster egg penetration
  - Computerized assessment of sperm motility
- Diagnostic IVF (see Section #30)

Principles of Management

Infected semen is treated with antibiotic therapy and, if indicated, prostatic massage. Pending culture and sensitivity testing, one of the following antibiotic regimens may be prescribed:

- Doxycycline at 100 mg bid for three weeks
- Ofloxacin at 300 mg bid for seven days
- Tetracycline at 500 mg qid for three weeks
- Erythromycin or ampicillin at 500 mg qid for three weeks

Hormonal therapy may be considered if levels are low, such as:

- Low LH:
  - HCG 250 units three times a week to 5,000 units three times a week, with:
    - Monitoring of plasma testosterone every two weeks AND
    - Semen analysis progress at six weekly intervals
- Low combined FSH and LH:
  - Clomiphene citrate at 25 to 50 mg daily for 25 out of 30 days in the month
  - HMG at one ampule two to three times a week for three to six months (for low to normal gonadotropins with poor motility and low testosterone)
  - Testosterone at 5 to 10 mg daily for three months

No pharmacological treatments are FDA-approved. Patients' hormonal blood work and semen analysis should be monitored frequently to facilitate early diagnosis and cessation of therapy for those in whom failure of stimulation or possible suppression of spermatogenesis are noted.

If sperm counts are greater than 10 million per mL with greater than 80 percent normal sperm and greater than 80 percent normal motility, further assessment of the female partner should be made.

Washed sperm intrauterine insemination (WIUI) treatments (see Section #28) may be attempted, using one of the following methods:

- Performed in the spontaneous cycle, with monitoring of LH surge
- By supplemented ovulation induction, with clomiphene citrate and/or HMG and HCG injection timed by ultrasound monitoring

The timing of WIUI treatments is crucial, since washed sperm survive for only a limited eight to 12 hours. Great precision is dictated in timing procedures as closely as possible to anticipated ovulation. This assessment may be made by:

- HCG administration
- Ultrasound monitoring
- Estradiol monitoring

#11 Hysterosalpingogram

Definition

The hysterosalpingogram (HSG) is an x-ray study of the inner female genital tract, which includes the:

- Cervix
- Uterus
- Fallopian tubes
- General pelvic status

The HSG should be completed soon after menstruation (approximately day eight of the menstrual cycle). However, it should not be performed if there is:

- Evidence of pelvic infection (chlamydia culture should be negative)
- Suggestion of pregnancy (if recent menses was abnormal, a negative pregnancy test is essential)

Prior to testing, a prophylactic antibiotic should be administered, eg, tetracycline at 500 g orally four times daily for five days, beginning one day before the procedure. Atropine at 0.4 to 1 mg IM should be administered 30 minutes before the procedure to reduce the likelihood of vasovagal reactions and to promote tubal relaxation.

Materials, Equipment and Instrumentation

Equipment necessary for HSG includes:

- Disposable plastic speculum
- Single-toothed tenaculum
- Rubber acorn cannula with an application end of no more than 3 mm beyond the tip of the rubber seal
- Multiple, long cotton sponges
- Betadine® preparation
- 20 percent benzocaine spray
- Water soluble medium (warmed)
- 20 cc disposable syringe

Clinical Procedure

The following criteria are essential for successful HSG:

- Adequate pelvic lighting
- Fluoroscopic monitoring

- Surgeon wearing lead apron
- Lead apron covering patient from buttocks to end of table (Figure 11.1)

A minimal number of pictures, preferably full pelvic films, should be completed.

The HSG progresses in sequential steps. To perform the HSG, the surgeon is to:

- Place the patient in the lithotomy position
- Insert the speculum and define the cervix
- Cleanse the cervix with Betadine®
- Dry the cervix with plain cotton bud
- Spray the cervix liberally with 20 percent benzocaine, wiping the excess from the posterior fornix with plain, dry cotton bud
- Cleanse the cervix again with Betadine®
- Grasp the cervix with a single-toothed tenaculum
- Check the fluid cannula to ensure that it is free of air bubbles; apply it with gentle countertraction
- Alert the radiologist
- Place the television monitor at patient's side so that it is visible to both doctors
- Load the x-ray plate into the fluoroscope screen, and draw it close to the patient to minimize magnification
- Pass the dye in small, two to three mL increments
- Take pictures at different positions (Figure 11.2), including:
    - Neutral position
    - Elevated position
    - Descensus position
- Take pictures at each position:
    - As the dye completes tubal filling
    - At early spill
    - With the spill occurring

  Once pictures are completed, a standing erect film at 20 minutes may be obtained in selected cases
- Remove the cannula and tenaculum under direct vision
- Use pressure to stop any tenaculum bleeding

- Place a tampon (with the tip soaked in Betadine®) in vagina and leave for two to three hours if indicated
- Immediately read the films with the radiologist
- Review the films with the patient

Documentation

The hysterosalpingogram will reveal:

- Uterine:
  - Site
  - Size
  - Lateral displacement (possible)
- Cervical canal
- Uterine fundus
- Cornual appearance
- Tubal:
  - Isthmus
  - Ampulla
  - Infundibulum
  - Fimbrial end
- Tubal mobility relative to uterine displacement
- Status of general pelvic spill
- Tubal endosalpingeal (mucosal) pattern
- Tubal saccular or general dilatation
- General tubal diameters, measured in comparison to size of the closed cervical tenaculum (1.2 cm)
- Spill pattern, ie, disseminated vs. loculated spill

Expectations of a normal HSG include:

- Central uterus which is mobile
- Narrow cervical canal
- Single, triangular, heart-shaped fundus
- Well-defined cornu, bilaterally
- Regular isthmus (some convolutions)
- Uniform ampulla with:
  - Symmetrical fill
  - Unhesitant spill
- Tubal movements during uterine:
  - Elevation
  - Descensus

- Rapid fill and spill in all directions
- Disseminated pelvic spill pattern with difficulty in defining "empty" tubes in erect, 20-minute film

The patient will experience minimal discomfort during the procedure.

Diagnostic Review/Possible Associations

Abnormalities noted at HSG and their possible causes may include:

- Extreme cervical narrowing caused by previous:
  - Coagulation
  - Cryosurgery
  - Laser surgery
  - Repeated dilatations
  - DES exposure
  - Recurrent cervicitis post-treatment
- Cervical incompetence associated with:
  - Funneling
  - Short cervical canal
  - Multiple cervical dilatations
  - Mid-trimester, painless miscarriage
  - Premature labor
  - Precipitate labor
  - DES exposure
  - Previous cervical cone biopsy

  If cervical incompetence is noted, there may be associated fundal uterine anomalies that are:
    - Septate
    - Bicornuate
    - Previous third-stage complications, such as retained placenta
    - Accreta
    - Increta
    - Percreta
- Cervical or isthmic extravasation caused by:
  - Previous caesarean section
  - Previous uterine perforation
  - Adenomyosis
- Vascular intravasation caused by:
  - Intrauterine synechiae
  - True proximal tubal occlusion

- Cervical pathology, including:
  - Polyps
  - Carcinomas
- Uterine cavity anomalies, including:
  - Congenital:
    - Arcuate
    - Septate
    - Bicornuate
    - Fundal, with cornual asymmetry disparity
  - Enlarged cavity
  - Small hypoplastic cavity
  - Variations (such as T-shaped)–Indication of DES exposure
  - Transfundal synechiae
  - Adenomyosis
  - Endometrial hyperplasia
  - Polyps or carcinomas
- Cornual area which is:
  - Widened or narrowed
  - Asymmetrical
  - Scarred
  - Polyped
  - Dilatated, indicating DES exposure
  - Spasmodic vs. occlusive:
    - True occlusion is evidenced by non-entry of dye contrast into interstitial oviduct
    - Commencement of dye entry into interstitium cannot be differentiated from spasm in a single HSG

    Spasm should be relieved by:
    - Warmed contrast
    - Adequate analgesic
    - Atropine
    - Glucagon
    - Gentle technique
- Isthmus which is:
  - Shortened
  - Elongated
  - Convoluted
  - Exhibiting diamond-shaped "lakes"–Indication of DES exposure

- Diverticular appearance, caused by:
  - Congenital anomalies
  - Endometriosis
  - Salpingitis isthmica nodosa
  - PID
  - Tuberculosis
- Ampullary segment that is:
  - Saccular dilatation and/or convolutions suggests:
    - Possible peritubal adhesions OR
    - Endometriosis
  - Distal narrowing, following widespread dilatation suggests:
    - Possible phimosis
  - Isthmo-ampullary and ampullary narrowing, showing a patchy, cotton-wool appearance of contrast caused by:
    - Severe PID
    - Tuberculosis
    - Rigid oviduct
- Distal tubal fixity, with no movement of isolated, often distorted segments, caused by possible peritubal adhesions
    - Tubes closed–Probable previous PID
    - Tubes open–Probable endometriosis
- Tubal occlusion:
  - Fair to good prognosis is anticipated (25 to 40 percent live births) with evidence of:
    - Multiple folds (rugal pattern)
    - Rapid emptying (of 20-minute film)
    - Minimal dilatation
    - Cartwheel appearance of distal oviduct
  - Poor outcome is anticipated (five to 25 percent live births) if:
    - No rugal folds are evident
    - There is a delay in emptying (still filled at 20-minute film)
    - Oviducts are dilated, large, flattened and smooth-walled
- Loculated spill, unilateral or bilateral, with limited dissemination of dye suggests peritubal adhesions

Principles of Management

See Section #22 for management protocols and Section #23 for classification of endometriosis.

If HSG is normal, supplemented ovulation induction should be begun and continued for approximately six months. The patient should be observed throughout the therapy.

Patients should consider hysteroscopy and laparoscopy as soon as feasible for:

- Tubal patency, but with possible:
  - Peritubal adhesions
  - Distortion
  - Endometriosis
  - Loculated spill
- Tubal occlusion or patency, but with marked dilatation and significantly delayed spill

Hysteroscopy and laparoscopy will ensure detailed uterine cavity assessment and evaluation of the overall pelvic peritoneal status.

FIGURE 11.1 – **Use of Lead Shielding at Hysterosalpingography**

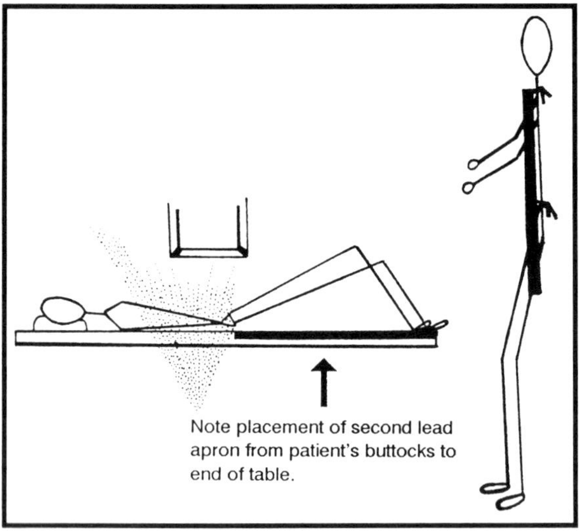

FIGURE 11.2—**Normal Series of Films at Hysterosalpingography**

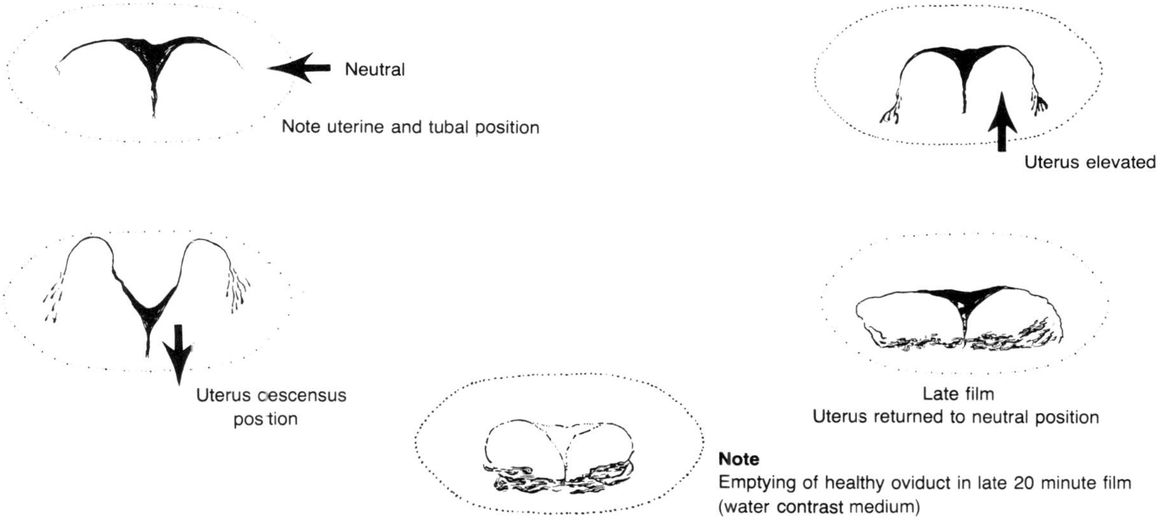

#12 Postcoital Test

Postcoital Evaluation and Timing of Ovulation

The postcoital test (PCT) provides evidence of adequate:

- Estrogen stimulation and mucus preparation of the female genital tract
- Mucus penetration by healthy, active spermatozoa

The PCT must be accurately timed and performed during the estrogen surge immediately prior to ovulation. It is usually completed:

- During cycle days 11 through 13
- When visible mucus is:
  - Adequate
  - Copious
  - Crystal-clear
- Within 24 hours of the LH surge, as detected by the urine LH surge guide
- When the estradiol (E_2) surge is observed (in patients monitored during ovulation induction)
- When an adequate, mature follicle is noted on ultrasound (18 to 25 mm) in association with the parameters listed above

Timing of the PCT

PCT evaluations may be completed within two, six, 12 or 18 hours of coitus. In healthy, normal, fertile patients, the PCT evaluation may be satisfactory even 36 and 48 hours after intercourse. If a PCT result is negative, a repeated test must be performed within two to six hours of intercourse in order to determine the precise numbers of motile sperm and the adequacy of sperm mucus penetration shortly after insemination.

The Normal PCT

The PCT is scheduled according to information derived from:

- The temperature graph (see Section #9)
- The menstrual calendar

- LH urine surge guide
- Hormonal (E_2) or ultrasound follicular data

For the most accurate results, the couple scheduled for a PCT should have intercourse within six hours of the examination, and the patient should not bathe, shower or douche prior to presentation at the office. It is recommended that the male partner have no knowledge of the impending test; such knowledge may cause performance stress which can negatively affect the ejaculate, sperm numbers and mucus penetration function.

Clinical Procedure

To perform the PCT, physicians are to:

- Place the patient in the lithotomy position
- Insert a vaginal speculum and visualize the cervix
- Wipe the cervix with a cotton bud
- Score the cervical mucus according to the Insler Scoring System (Table 12.1)

TABLE 12.1 – **Insler Scoring System for Cervical Mucus (Maximal "Perfect" Score = 12)**

	Trace	**Moderate**	**Copious**
Amount	+	++	+++
Spinnbarkeit	0 to 2 cms	3 to 6 cms	> 8 cms
Ferning	Trace and single branches	Moderate double branches	Total with multiple branches
Cervical Os	Slightly open	Moderately open	Patulous

Documentation

The status of the cervix is documented according to:

- Amount of mucus
- Quality of spinnbarkeit
- Degree of opening
- Presence of ferning
- Clarity of mucus vs. presence of cellular debris or leukocytes

This documentation indicates correct timing and normal receptivity conditions.

To prepare the sample for documentation, physicians are to:

- Aspirate the samples of cervical mucus from the cervical canal with a sterile tuberculin syringe
- Apply gentle suction and withdraw the syringe while dividing the mucus column with a forceps to withdraw the secretion
- Place the secretion on a warm slide and cover with a cover slip
- Incubate the slide at body temperature and evaluate (Figure 12.1)

Initially, a panoramic view of the total field and impression of the concentration of spermatozoa is performed. Then individual sperm are assessed for:

- Numbers
- Motility
- Speed of forward progression

The slide is then viewed under high power and documented for:

- Number of sperm per high power field
- Speed of forward progression (indicated on a scale of 0 to 4)

In a healthy, fertile couple, it is impossible to count the number of sperm per high power field (hundreds); the forward progression speed will range from two to four.

Classically, more than 20 sperm per high power field with excellent speed of forward progression is compatible with fertility, but 15 to 20 sperm are also likely to be compatible. Pregnancies have occurred at rates of only five active sperm per high power field at the mid-cycle PCT evaluation.

Figure 12.2 illustrates possible results found in PCT slide samples of donor crossmatch testing performed to determine causes of infertility related to cervical mucus factors or spermatozoa penetration insufficiency (see Section #24).

Figures 12.1 and 12.2 ➡

FIGURE 12.1 — **Aspiration of Cervical Mucus During Postcoital Test**

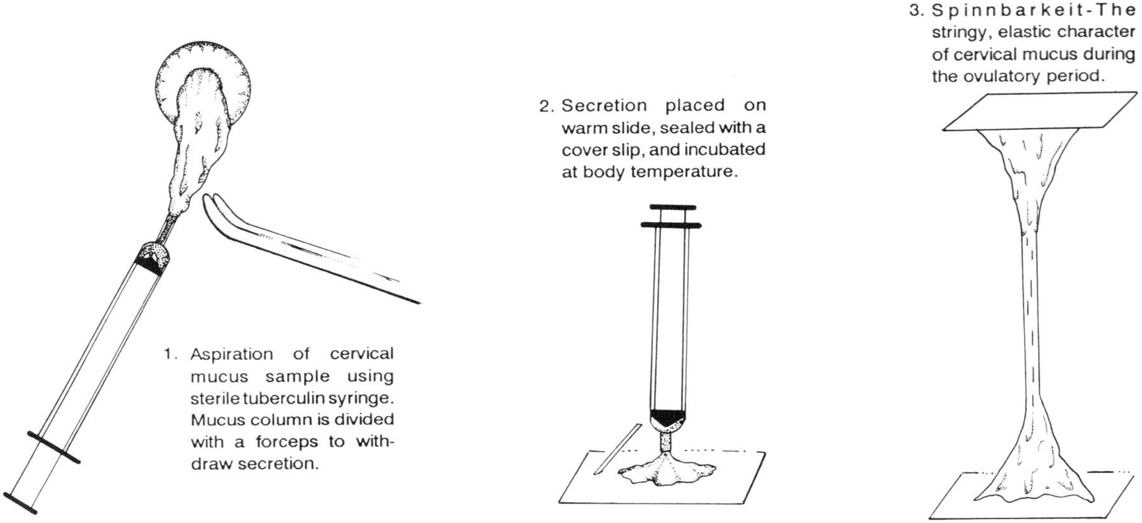

4. Panoramic view of slide sample.

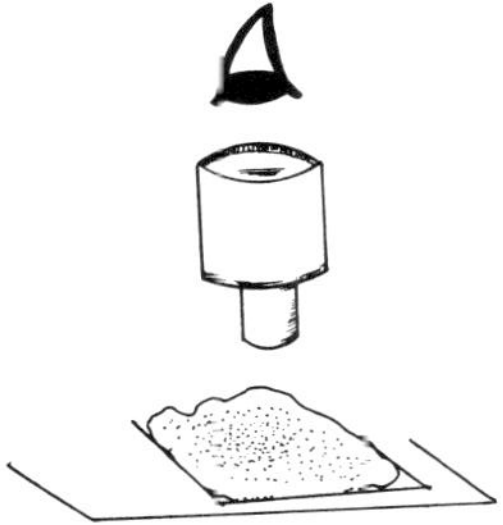

5. Scan for numbers, motility and speed of forward progression of sperm.

6. High power view—Documentation of number of sperm per high power field.

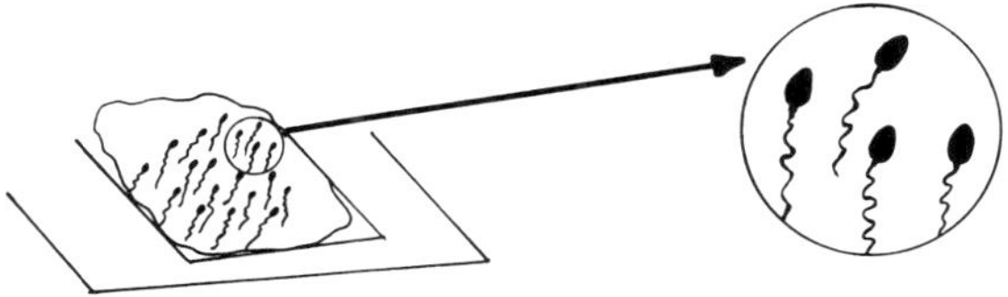

FIGURE 12.2 — **Donor Mucus and Sperm Crossmatch Testing — Evaluation of Mucus/Sperm Failure of Penetration**

General Appearances of Mucus/Sperm Penetration	Female Mucus — Cause of Abnormality	Male Spermatozoa — Cause of Abnormality
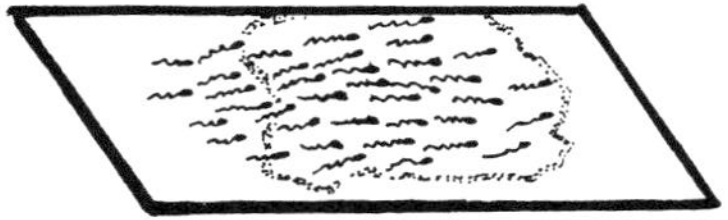	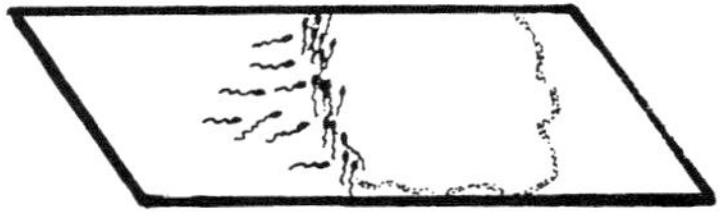	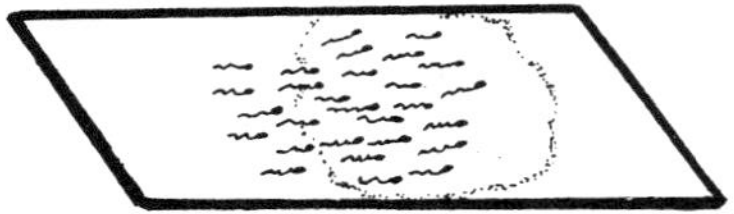
Sperm: Husband — Mucus: Wife NORMAL True penetration.	Sperm: Donor — Mucus: Wife ABNORMAL Suspect problem with mucus.	Sperm: Donor — Mucus: Wife NORMAL Suspect problem with sperm.
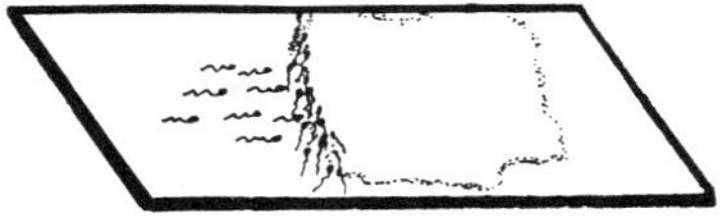	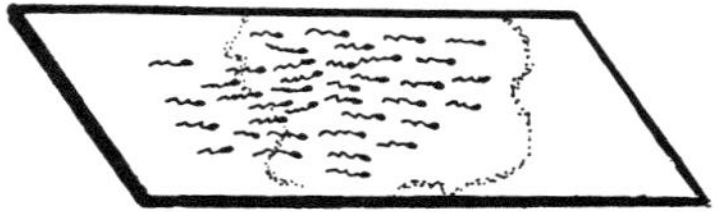	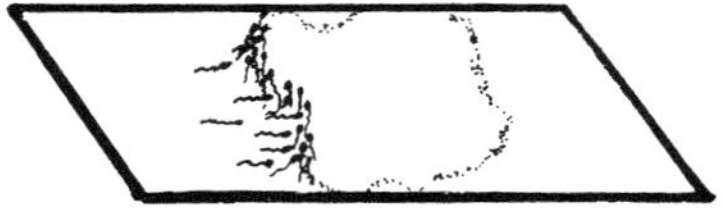
Sperm: Husband — Mucus: Wife ABNORMAL No penetration.	Sperm: Husband — Mucus: Donor NORMAL Confirms problem with mucus.	Sperm: Husband — Mucus: Donor ABNORMAL Confirms problem with sperm.

NOTES

#13 Hormonal Testing: Male and Female

MALE

Hormone Evaluation

To determine causes of infertility relating to the male factor, an evaluation should be made of:

- Testosterone
- FSH
- LH
- Prolactin
- TSH, T_3 and T_4
- Estradiol (if indicated)

In the male, lack of libido may be associated with low plasma testosterone and/or hyperprolactinemia. A low testosterone level may be secondary to either testicular failure or inadequate hypothalamic-pituitary-gonadal stimulation. Abnormally high levels of estrogen may be linked to liver dysfunction and/or chronic liver damage.

Low testosterone may be due to the absence of testicular stimulation by gonadotropins. Low gonadotropins (FSH and LH) combined with low testosterone indicate hypogonadotropic hypogonadism. Testicular biopsy will reveal testicular tissue with arrest of spermatogenesis but with a healthy and abundant germinal epithelium. This patient should be referred to an urologist and treated with human menopausal gonadotropins (HMG) of 1 ampule two to three times a week for at least six to 10 weeks and human chorionic gonadotropin (HCG) at 2,000 units three times a week as maintenance therapy.

Normal testicular biopsy associated with low pituitary gonadotropins or low FSH:LH ratio may be evidence of inadequate stimulation of Leydig's cells (testosterone production) due to the low LH. To affect normalization of spermatogenesis, LH should be administered as HCG in small-dose injections of 250 to 2,000 IU three times a week to elevate testosterone production.

Gonadal failure is evidenced by high FSH and LH. In these cases, the gonadal biopsy will be associated with evidence of testicular failure. FSH measurements in the 30 to 50 range commonly confirm gonadal failure. There is no treatment protocol in these circumstances, though androgen replacement therapy may be given to maintain normal sexual function.

Elevated prolactin may be associated with other pituitary abnormalities, including acromegaly and/or Cushing's syndrome. Pituitary neoplasms are excluded by CAT scan or nuclear magnetic resonance imaging (MRI).

If tests reveal hyperprolactinemia, the patient is treated with bromocriptine, beginning with a dose of 2.5 mg hs and increasing the dosage every five to seven days until normal levels are established. Caution is advised in the initial administration of this agent due to the possibility of hypotensive side effects. Patients are encouraged to take their pills at bedtime and to consume increased amounts of fluids during therapy.

In all instances, repeat assays of plasma testosterone should be conducted at three week intervals, and follow-up semen analysis should be performed and reviewed 60 days after therapy commences.

In some cases, down regulation of receptors may occur with an associated fall in testosterone and further deterioration demonstrated by semen analysis. This is usually temporary but emphasizes the need for cautious monitoring during the administration of any medications.

CAVEAT: Not all therapeutic options for males have current FDA approval. Therefore, patients should be fully advised by their clinicians regarding the rationale for choosing specific options.

FEMALE

Hormone Evaluation

Hormonal tests for women should evaluate:

- Pituitary gonadotropins
  - FSH
  - LH

- Prolactin
- Thyroid
  - TSH, T_3 and T_4
  - Thyroid uptake
  - Free thyroxine index (FTI)
- Adrenal
  - Cortisol
  - Dehydroepiandrosterone sulphate (DHEAS)
  - Androstenedione
  - 17-hydroxyprogesterone
- Ovary
  - Estradiol
  - Estrone
  - Testosterone

In patients presenting with normal body weight and a regular 28-day menstrual cycle (see Section #2), hormonal testing should reveal physiological normals as follows:

- Gonadotropins:
  - FSH – 5 to 15 mIU/mL
  - LH – 5 to 15 mIU/mL
- Prolactin – 3 to 20 ng/mL
- Thyroid uptake:
  - TSH – Less than 5 μIU/mL
  - T_3 – 80 to 200 ng/dL
  - T_4 – 4 or 5 to 13 μg/dL
- Adrenal:
  - Plasma cortisol – 5 to 15 mg/dL, with morning and evening variations:
    - Maximum level at approximately 10:00 a.m.
    - Minimum level at approximately 4:00 p.m.
  - DHEAS – 0.5 to 2.5 mcg/mL
- Ovary:
  - Estradiol:
    - Early proliferative phase – 20 to 60 pg/mL
    - Mid-cycle late proliferative phase – 80 to 250 pg/mL
    - Luteal phase – 60 to 120 pg/mL
  - Plasma testosterone – 20 to 80 ng/mL

Clinical Presentations/Associations

Conditions associated with infertility include:

- Dysovulatory
  - Amenorrhea
  - Oligomenorrhea
  - Menstrual dysfunction
  - Prolonged or short follicular/proliferative phase
  - Short luteal phase–Indication of variations in secretory/luteal phase defects
- Weight and eating disorders
  - Thin body habitus
  - Anorexic
  - Previous major weight gain or loss
  - Obesity
- Changing body habitus
  - Cushingoid facies
- Hypothalamic-pituitary
  - Recurrent severe headaches
  - Visual field defects
  - Head injury, previous coma, loss of consciousness
  - Persistent stress

  These dysfunctions are usually experienced by compulsive athletes, ballerinas, joggers or gymnasts
- Androgen dysfunction–Indication of adrenal or gonadal hyperandrogenism
  - Hirsutism
  - Virilization
- Thyroid
  - Galactorrhea
  - Sluggishness
  - Cold intolerance
  - Pretibial edema
  - Voice changes
- Metabolic
  - Diabetes
  - Polydypsia, polyphagia and polyuria
  - Dizzy spells
  - Cold sweats

Physical Examination

Examination of body habitus should reveal:

- Thin vs. fat
- Hirsutism
  - Virilized over the beard and chest area
  - Balding
- Perianal hirsutism with an excess of hair on back
- Cushingoid buffalo hump
- Vaginal dryness vs. moistness
- Cervix with estrogen "turned off" vs. "switched on"
  - "Turned off" causes cervical dryness
  - "Switched on" indicates a cervix which is well-estrogenized and has abundant, clear mucus
- Uterus which is clinically small vs. normal
- Ovaries which are quiescent vs. large and polycystic as determined by palpation or vaginal ultrasound
- Visual field defects
- Possible premature menopause
- Decreased vs. increased libido

Assessment

The hypoestrogenic patient may have hypogonadotropic hypogonadism (common in hypothalamic pituitary amenorrhea with low or barely recordable gonadotropins).

The patient with ovarian failure is indicated by:

- Low estrogen
- Elevated gonadotropins with FSH greater than 40 on two occasions assessed three to six weeks apart (this is suggestive of menopause)

If hyperprolactinemia is revealed, further assessment of pituitary status by either CAT scan or MRI as a baseline is indicated. Causes to be excluded include:

- Pregnancy
- Drug ingestion
  - Sedatives
  - Hypnotics
  - Narcotics

- Stress
- Previous chest injury
- Breast stimulation
- Hypothyroidism
- Pituitary microadenoma or adenomatous hyperplasia

Treatment is essentially the same as for ovulatory disorders using bromocriptine (see Section #20).

Hypothalamic Amenorrhea

Diagnosis of hypothalamic amenorrhea is indicated by:

- Thinness
- Low body weight
- Stress
- Athletic activity
- Eating disorders
- Anorexia
- Bulimia
- Associated hyperandrogenism (possibly)
- Associated low to normal thyroid and adrenal functions, together with low to normal plasma androgens

The diagnosis is made by physical examination which should reveal:

- Low body weight
- Low body fat
- Sparse hair (lanugo)
- Decreased breast tissue
- Vaginal examination showing relative dryness and atrophy; hypoestrogenic cervical mucus will be dry–Indication of small pelvic organs and small, inactive ovaries (these can be confirmed by ultrasound)

Additionally, a progesterone challenge test should be performed by administering 10 mg of medroxyprogesterone acetate (MPA) for five days. If test is negative, the patient will not menstruate after withdrawal of MPA.

Diagnosis is confirmed by low gonadotropins (FSH and LH at 0 to 5). If bleeding occurs (meaning a positive progesterone challenge test), the presence of prior basal, normal estrogen function is confirmed.

Principles of Management

Hypothalamic Amenorrhea

If possible, the cause of the hormonal dysfunction must be removed and the patient counseled regarding:

- Diet
- Stress
- Athletic pursuits
- Weight gain (indicating need for nutritional counseling)
- Estrogen/progesterone maintenance therapy (conjugated estrogens 0.625 mg daily for cycle days one through 25 and MPA 10 mg daily for cycle days 13 to 25) to prevent:
  - Osteoporosis
  - Atherogenesis

Ovulation induction with HMG may treat ovulatory disorders (see Section #20) resulting from hypothalamic pituitary dysfunction.

Premature Menopause

Patients complaining of hot flashes may be experiencing premature menopause. To confirm this, a general examination will reveal:

- Hypoestrogenic status
- Vaginal dryness and atrophy
- Absence of cervical mucus
- Elevated gonadotropins (FSH and LH greater than 40 mIU/mL on two occasions)
- Associated features of an autoimmune disorder or abnormal thyroid function

In general, the prognosis for premature menopause is poor. The patient may be offered estrogen replacement therapy and subsequent withdrawal, and this may result in rebound ovulation and conception.

Treatment may also consist of:

- Estrogen preparations, such as conjugated estrogens at 1.25 mg daily for 25 days
- MPA at 5 mg daily for five days (cycle days 21 through 25) followed by:
  - HMG trial, with assessment of estradiol from the fifth day, to assess a positive response of residual follicles (indicated by rising estradiol levels)

All patients must have karyotype to exclude an associated Y chromosome. The presence of a Y chromosome indicates the need for gonadectomy to prevent subsequent ovarian malignancy.

Possible laparoscopy and ovarian biopsy is considered an invasive means of assessing residual oocytes in the gonad; furthermore, a single ovarian biopsy may not be representative of the total gonadal tissue.

Thyroid Status

HYPERTHYROIDISM

Hyperthyroidism is indicated by:

- Elevated T_3 and T_4
- Low TSH
- Associated weight loss
- Agitation
- Vasodilatation which is well perfused
- Associated palpitations
- Possible intermittent dyspnea

On examination, hyperthyroidism will show:

- Tremor
- Exophthalmos
- Eyelid retraction
- Tachycardia
- Muscle irritability

The patient may need to be referred for endocrine studies and/or surgical consultation. Treatment may consist of:

- Antithyroid preparations
- Radioactive sodium iodine
- Thyroidectomy

Subsequent assessment of ovulation and ovulation induction with correction of luteal phase defect should follow treatment, if applicable.

HYPOTHYROIDISM

Hypothyroidism is seen in a significant number of patients, especially when present in the family history. Early onset is subtle, but symptoms include:

- Tiredness
- Lack of energy
- Weight gain and/or pretibial edema
- Intolerance of cold environments
- Persistent feelings of coldness
- Voice changes
- Depression

Noted on examination are:

- Obesity
- Relatively slow mannerism
- Possible goiter
- Dryness of skin
- Absence of hair
- Pretibial edema

The earliest evidence of hypothyroidism is elevated thyroid-stimulating hormone (TSH). Since TSH can be elevated while the thyroid maintains adequate hormone production because of elevated TSH stimulation, T_3 and T_4 may be normal. A thyrotropin-releasing hormone (TRH) stimulation test may be indicated. In this test, TRH is administered and measurements of TSH are taken immediately and at intervals of:

- 15 minutes
- 30 minutes
- One hour
- One and one-half hours

Elevated basal TSH indicates a positive test result; a massive rise occurs in hypothyroidism. If the TSH level change is minimal, the patient is euthyroid.

Managing hypothyroidism includes:

- Administration of synthyroid, a synthetic thyroid preparation, at an average dosage of 0.05 mg per day
- Monitoring of TSH, which should return to less than 5 mIU with therapy

Adrenal Hyperandrogenism

Adrenal hyperandrogenism is indicated by elevated DHEAS. Management involves the assessment of 17-hydroxyprogesterone to diagnose possible enzyme defect (21/23 hydroxylase).

Treatment includes administration of corticosteroids, such as dexamethasone 0.5 mg hs (with a snack as a precaution to avoid gastric ulceration), supplemented with clomiphene citrate (to induce ovulation).

Treatment to induce ovulation using dexmethasone in combination with clomiphene citrate rather than clomiphene citrate alone results in more successful ovulations and pregnancies, once DHEAS is greater than 200 ng/dL.

True adrenogenital syndrome is treated with the administration of corticosteroids while monitoring androgens. Once androgens are in a normal range, patients usually ovulate normally.

An adrenal tumor, indicated by extremely high levels of DHEAS, should be excluded by a dexamethasone suppression test. For the test, the patient is to take 1 mg of dexamethasone at 11:00 p.m. on the evening before the test. Blood is to be drawn at 8:00 a.m. on the following morning and the sample observed. Dexamethasone suppression and the absence of an adrenal tumor is indicated by a drop in plasma cortisol overnight. A level of less than 5 ng/dL excludes Cushing's syndrome.

Ovarian Hyperandrogenism and Elevated Plasma Testosterone

Ovarian hyperandrogenism and elevated plasma testosterone most commonly present as polycystic ovarian syndrome (PCO). Occasionally this results from:

- Stromal hyperplasia
- Hilar cell hyperplasia
- Testosterone-producing ovarian tumors (eg, Leydig's cell tumor or arrhenoblastoma)

With PCO, an elevation in the LH to FSH ratio is common, but an ovarian tumor should be excluded if plasma testosterone is greater than 200 ng/dL. Combination estrogen/progestin pills (oral contraceptives [OCs]) are used for 25 to 30 days as a diagnostic measure, after which plasma levels are re-measured. A significant drop in testosterone indicates ovarian dysfunction and excludes a tumor.

An association exists between ovarian hyperandrogenism and miscarriage following ovulation induction. In the presence of elevated androgens, this indicates the need to suppress the ovarian androgen output with OCs before beginning ovulation induction therapy.

Treatment includes:

- Clomiphene citrate at a starting dose of 50 mg and adding dexamethasone at 0.5 mg; this is to be taken at night if the ovarian hyperandrogenism is associated with elevated DHEAS levels
- Bromocriptine, if the ovarian hyperandrogenism is associated with hyperprolactinemia
- GnRH agonists

Protocol for ovulation induction (see Section #20) includes:

- Clomiphene citrate plus HCG OR
- HMG (possibly) and/or pure FSH plus HCG

NOTE: The physician should exclude any negative cervical factor and/or luteal phase deficiency when using clomiphene citrate in large doses or for prolonged periods of time.

Hypercortisolism

Primary pituitary vs. primary adrenal causes must be assessed (Cushing's syndrome vs. Cushing's disease).

Hypercortisolism requires therapy with cortisone suppression (dexamethasone), subsequent assessment of adequate ovulatory function and/or use of ovulation induction with clomiphene citrate plus HCG and possible progesterone suppositories (see Section #20).

#14 Plasma Progesterone and Endometrial Biopsy

Definition

Plasma progesterone and endometrial biopsy facilitate assessment of the quality of ovulation. The mid-luteal phase progesterone (occurring approximately six to seven days after ovulation) should correspond to the optimal production of progesterone by the corpus luteum.

Data may be reviewed as follows:

- Morning samples of plasma progesterone should be greater than 5 ng/mL
- Plasma progesterones less than 10 ng/mL are commonly associated with luteal phase defects and/or short luteal phases
- Three random plasma progesterones taken in the luteal phase should be cumulatively greater than 15 ng/mL

The mid-luteal plasma progesterone result may be used as a screening parameter. If it is less than 10 ng/mL, endometrial biopsy will most likely be compatible with luteal phase defect. If greater than 10 ng/mL, a timed luteal phase endometrial biopsy on cycle day 26 or later should be obtained to corroborate the adequacy of the luteal phase.

Endometrial biopsy is not completed if the progesterone is less than 10 ng/mL. Instead, correction of the level and assessment of the luteal phase adequacy by timed endometrial biopsy is attempted.

A plasma progesterone level of less than 2 ng/mL indicates an anovulatory cycle.

The Endometrial Biopsy

The endometrial biopsy provides a "bioassay" of the adequacy of endometrial estrogen and progesterone preparation and receptivity of the endometrium to morula or blastocyst implantation. In view of the discrepancy of interpretations by different pathologists at different stages of the menstrual cycle, the biopsy is best completed at or after cycle day 26, when final maturation of the endometrium is easily confirmed. By this time, the endometrium has achieved:

- Minimal glandular activity
- Adequate stromal swelling
- Deciduation
- Leukocytic infiltration
- Perivascular cellular activity

Earlier in the cycle (ie, days 21 through 23), pathological interpretation is confusing and more difficult, since variations in endometrial preparation are greater at this stage.

The biopsy is always interpreted relative to the next menstrual cycle; the days are counted backwards, days 28, 27, etc. For patients with a 35-day menstrual cycle, for example, day 35 would correspond to day one, day 34 to day 28, day 33 to day 27, etc.

Indications for Endometrial Biopsy

The biopsy is timed for day 26 of the menstrual cycle, 10 days or more after the temperature change or 12 days or more after the LH surge and/or administration of HCG at mid-cycle.

Indications for biopsy include:

- A short luteal phase (less than 10 days postovulation)
- Normal to low plasma progesterones are present with suspect variations in the temperature graph (eg, a slow rise over five or six days postovulation or a low rise of 0.4 as opposed to greater than 0.6 degrees F)
- A temperature rise which subsequently falls early in the normal luteal phase
- Clomiphene citrate therapy for ovarian stimulation
- Treatment for hyperprolactinemia
- Previous documented hyperandrogenism (ie, elevated plasma testosterone or adrenal DHEAS)
- HMG therapy
- Recurrent prolonged proliferative phases

Clinical Procedure

Physicians must obtain a negative quantitative βHCG within 24 hours of the test. At the patient's arrival, he should check the status of ovulation on the temperature graph or recent plasma progesterone, together with the negative βHCG. If no contraindications are present, the endometrial biopsy may be performed.

The clinical procedure for endometrial biopsy is to:

- Administer atropine 0.4 mg IM 20 to 30 minutes before the procedure
- Place the patient in the lithotomy position
- Perform a pelvic examination to confirm the status and position of the uterus
- Define the cervix with a speculum
- Dry the cervix with a cotton sponge, and spray it with a 20-percent benzocaine solution
- Cleanse the cervix with Betadine®, and apply a benzocaine solution to the cervical canal, using a sterile cotton swab
- Cleanse the cervix once more with Betadine®
- After informing the patient of the procedure, grasp the cervix with a single-toothed tenaculum
- Pass a disposable, plastic cannula through the cervical canal to the uterine fundus, and withdraw the inner plunger to create suction and obtain a fine endometrial biopsy
    - If this method fails to produce an adequate biopsy, insert a Novak curette through the cervical canal to complete the biopsy
- When the biopsy is completed, withdraw the vaginal instruments and remove the speculum
- Place the biopsy directly in formalin
- Submit the biopsy for histology
- Have the patient lie quietly for a few minutes following the procedure
- Instruct the patient to contact the clinic on the first day of bleeding (day one); compare this date to the biopsy report, using the criteria of Noyes, Hertig, and Rock (see Section #5, Figure 5.2)

Principles of Management

Management of abnormal endometrial biopsy (luteal phase defect) involves the diagnosis and treatment of all aberrations of adequate:

- Follicular maturation
- Mid-cycle LH surge
- Corpus luteum progesterone production (see Section #20)

Options include:

- Correction of hyperprolactinemia
- Correction of hyperandrogenism
- Progesterone vaginal suppositories
- HCG
- Clomiphene citrate with HCG
- HMG, HCG and progesterone suppositories (see Section #20)

#15 Hysteroscopy

Definition

Hysteroscopy is the examination of the inner uterus via an endoscope. This procedure is commonly completed at the time of laparoscopy to facilitate monitoring of operative hysteroscopy (see Section #27).

The objectives of hysteroscopy include:

- Assessment of the uterine cavity
- Assessment of endometrium
- A detailed examination of tubal cornu
- The exclusion of:
  - Fundal abnormalities
  - Intrauterine polyps
  - Intrauterine scarring (synechiae)
  - Possible intracavitary tumors (benign or malignant)
  - Chronic infection

Where pathology is present, hysteroscopy allows for possible:

- Operative endoscopy
- Transection of septum
- Division of synechiae
- Removal of polyps
- Selective biopsy

New techniques of hysteroscopy (Figure 15.1) include:

- Endometrial ablation
- Removal of proximal tubal obstructions by catheterization of tubal ostium at cornu
- Passage of gametes into oviduct via uterine cornu

Clinical Procedure

For the hysteroscopy, the physician is to:

- Place the patient in the lithotomy position
- Perform a pelvic examination to confirm uterine:
  - Size
  - Position
  - Mobility
- Insert a speculum and view the cervix

- Grasp the cervix with a single-toothed tenaculum
- Sound the uterus
- Dilate the cervix to one diameter less than the endoscope (hysteroscope) being used (eg, H-3 for 4 mm scope or H-5 for 6 mm scope)
- Insert the hysteroscope, with CO_2 or a distension medium flowing (see below)
- Visualize the cervical canal and enter
- Explore the uterine cavity systematically, being sure to include:
  - Right wall
  - Right cornu
  - Fundus
  - Left cornu
  - Left wall
  - Anterior wall
  - Posterior wall
  - Cervical canal (upon withdrawal)
- Withdraw instruments
- Document findings

Hysteroscopic Media

Distending media options include:

- CO_2 from hysteroflater, with:
  - Low volume flow of 20 to 60 mL per minute
  - High pressures of 10 to 100 mm Hg
- D5W
- Normal saline (contraindicated with electrocoagulation)
- Ringer's lactate (contraindicated with electrocoagulation)
- High molecular weight (70,000) dextran (Hyskon®) – CO_2 is preferred for diagnostic work but is not practical once bleeding occurs

Media for operative hysteroscopy include:

- Sorbitol
- D5 or D10 (with electrocoagulation)
- Ringer's lactate or normal saline, with:
  - High volume
  - High pressure irrigation (for distension)

By using these media, instrument cleaning problems are avoided and patients are at minimal risk if the substances are absorbed systemically. With the exception of D5 and D10, these media are contraindicated with electrocoagulation.

Although high molecular weight dextran is an ideal medium for operative endoscopy once bleeding occurs, associated problems may result from its use, including:

- Risk of fluid overload, including pulmonary edema if dextran is absorbed systemically
- Risk of:
  - Allergic reactions
  - DIC
  - Cardiopulmonary reactions
- Cleansing problems, because of the need for wide-bore installation scopes. Immediate post-use cleansing is urged to avoid the stickiness and sealing of joints, tubes and on/off valves

Documentation

Surgeons must document their findings, via diagrams, etc., immediately following the hysteroscopic examination. If abnormalities are noted, the physician should proceed with hysteroscopic correction, most commonly done in association with laparoscopic monitoring (see Section #16).

Many procedures are accomplished by working directly from video monitoring.

FIGURE 15.1 – **Principles of Hysterscopy**

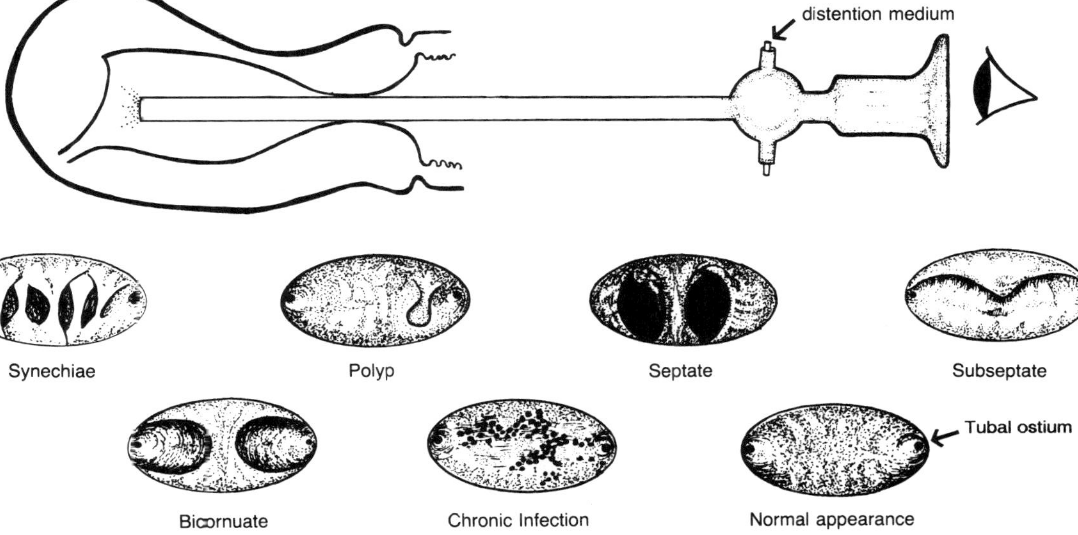

		CENTER
1.	Hypothalamic-Pituitary-Gonadal Function in the Male	Anatomy And Physiology of Conception
2.	Hypothalamic-Pituitary-Gonadal Function in the Female	
3.	Menstrual Cycle: Response of Female Genital Tract	
4.	Sperm Cycle in Female	
5.	Ovulation, Fertilization and Postovulatory Events	
6.	Clinicopathological Factors	
7.	Primary Consultation: History and Physical	Overview of Fertility Evaluation/ Management
8.	Planning of Investigation and Treatment	
9.	The Temperature Graph	Diagnostic Tests/ Treatment
10.	Semen Analysis	
11.	Hysterosalpingogram	
12.	Postcoital Test	
13.	Hormonal Testing: Male and Female	
14.	Plasma Progesterone and Endometrial Biopsy	
15.	Hysteroscopy	

INDEX

#16 Laparoscopy

Definition

Laparoscopy is used for endoscopic assessment of the pelvis to determine possible mechanical causes of infertility and to diagnose endometriosis. The laparoscope provides for panoramic assessment of:

- Pelvis
- Uterus
- Fallopian tubes
- Ovaries
- Tubo-ovarian relationships

The procedure involves the systematic observation of:

- Anterior vesicouterine peritoneum
- Rectosigmoid-pelvic relationships
- Peritoneum of the pelvic sidewalls, including ovarian fossae
- Tubal status and patency (by chromotubation)
- The status of the:
  - Cornu
  - Isthmus
  - Ampulla
  - Fimbria
  - Tubal ostium
- The status of fimbria ovarica and the proximity of the tubal ostium to ovarian surface (should be one to two cms in length) (Figure 16.1)

Laparoscopy will reveal the presence of any adhesions and their:

- Site
- Nature:
  - Flimsy vs. fibrosed
  - Ischemic vs. vascular

These findings are to be documented according to classifications of the American Fertility Society (Figure 16.2 and Figure 16.3).

Also to be documented from the procedure are the free flow and dispersed fimbriae in pelvic fluid vs.:

- Distal tubal stenosis
- Phimosis

- Agglutination of fimbriae
- Distal tubal dilatation
- Peritoneal lesions (which may require biopsy)

Postoperative Methodology

Laparoscopy should be performed during the mid-proliferative phase of the menstrual cycle. (It can be performed on day 26 of a 28-day cycle at the time of an endometrial biopsy if βHCG is negative [see Section #14]).

Physicians should determine preoperatively that no pelvic inflammatory disease (PID) exists or is suspected. The sedimentation rate should be normal and cervical cultures should be negative for:

- Chlamydia
- Mycoplasma
- Ureaplasma
- Neisseria gonorrhoeae

A normal EKG should be obtained, and blood studies should be performed for CBC and SMAC.

Patients should be instructed not to ingest any food or drink after midnight of the evening preceding the operation.

The surgery is commonly performed using general anesthesia with tracheal intubation. Total relaxation of the patient promotes safety by preventing sudden coughing or movements of internal viscera during insertion of the Verres needle or trocar and cannula.

Accurate readings should be maintained on pressure meters during needle penetration and subsequent gas insufflation. Pressures should be maintained below 14 mm Hg to avoid significant reduction of venous return by vena caval compression.

During surgery, adequate monitoring should be maintained for:

- Vital signs
- EKG
- pO_2
- pCO_2

Ventilation and fluid management should be sustained as indicated by the monitored cardiovascular changes.

Clinical Procedure

To perform the laparoscopy, surgeons are to:

- Drain the patient's bladder
- Place the patient in the lithotomy position
- Perform a pelvic examination
- Sound the uterus, and document its length
- Complete a hysteroscopy, if indicated (see Section #15)
- Insert the cervical cannula and attach it to the cervical tenaculum for connection to a sterile 60 mL syringe
- Use indigo carmine for subsequent dye injection to confirm tubal patency
- Carefully palpate the abdomen and assess the site of umbilicus relative to sacral promontory
- Compress the stomach area as the anesthesiologist inserts the nasogastric tube; suction to prevent gastric distention
- Prepare and drape the abdomen
- Ensure that lighting is perfect; this is essential
- Define the umbilicus, retract inferiorly and make a small incision (Figure 16.4)
- Insert the Verres needle through the incision, "feeling" passage through the fascia and the "pop" of penetrating the peritoneum
- Check the needle for free flow of fluid with 5 cc syringe of saline solution
- Check basal pressures, with the insufflator on automatic and in the on and off positions
- Once pressures are correct, switch the insufflator to manual. Pressures should remain at 0 to 10 mm mercury, with free flow
- Repeat a pressure check at the on and off positions
- Insufflate approximately three to four liters of carbon dioxide until adequate distension and pressures are attained (12 to 14 mm mercury)
- Insert trocar and cannula, with skin and anterior abdominal wall elevated, while assistant pulls uterus downward

- Attach a light cable, and insert the laparoscope
- Return the insufflator to automatic mode, and reattach to cannula
- Insert the second and/or third probe trocars and cannulas after:
  - Definition of anterior abdominal blood vessels in darkness
  - Observation through laparoscope during abdominal entry
- When the procedure is completed, pass abundant fluids through the oviducts at chromotubation and suction from the cul-de-sac
- Make a final check for potential organ injury and perfect hemostasis
- Withdraw all instruments
- Exsufflate all gas to reduce postoperative pain
- Suture the incision subcutaneously and apply steri-strips to the skin
- Remove vaginal instruments
- Check carefully for hemostasis at the site of the tenaculum
- Immediately document and diagram all findings

Examination

The laparoscope will reveal:

- General pelvic panorama
- Presence or absence of pelvic fluid
- Possible endometriosis
- Possible adhesions

For the examination, physicians are to:

- Aspirate pelvic fluids for culture and cytology examination
- Document endometriosis (if discovered), along with any adhesions, using AFS classifications (Figures 16.2 and 16.3)
- Assess all peritoneal surfaces, including:
  - Anterior
  - Posterior
  - Lateral

- Broad ligament:
  - Anterior
  - Posterior
- Elevate the ovaries and assess ovarian fossae
- Elevate the fallopian tubes and examine from uterus to fimbrial ends to reveal:
  - Fimbrial status:
    - Widely opened
    - Partially narrowed
    - Interfimbrial adhesions
  - True phimosis
    - Dilation of distal ampulla
    - Total occlusion
  - Small hydrosalpinges (less than one cm dilatation):
    - Well vascularized
    - Fibrosed
    - Ischemic
  - Medium hydrosalpinges (less than two cms dilatation):
    - Vascular
    - Ischemic
  - Large hydrosalpinges (greater than two cms dilatation):
    - Vascular
    - Ischemic
- Assess the relationship of the fallopian tubes to the ovaries, including:
  - Peritubal adhesions:
    - Thin, fibrosed
    - Thick, vascular
  - Parovarian cysts
  - Proximity of tubal ostium to ovarian surface:
    - Close vs. distant
  - Measurement of fimbria ovarica; document length as assessed by second-probe cm scale:
    - Less than two cms
    - Two to four cms
    - Greater than four cms

- Assessment of chromotubation:
  - Bilateral rapid fill and spill
  - Unilateral delay or occlusion

Documentation

The laparoscopy will reveal:

- Ovarian:
  - Site
  - Size
  - Shape
- Functional assessment of:
  - Follicular activity
  - Corpus luteum, ie, fresh or old

If pathology is present and is operable laparoscopically, the surgeon may proceed to operative laparoscopy (see Section #27); such cases include:

- Salpingolysis
- Ovariolysis
- Laser vaporization of endometriosis
- Laser drainage and vaporization of selected endometriomas
- Drainage and biopsy of ovarian cysts
- Selected salpingoneostomy

Ancillary Methods

Auxiliary methods of recording laparoscopic findings may be used, including:

- Photo documentation
- 35 mm color slides
- 35 mm Polaroid® photographs
- Video recordings
- Printouts of photographs selected from video camera
- Video or laser laparoscopy (see Section #27)

Patient Counseling

Physicians should compile all documented data from fertility testing, including results of:

- HSG (see Section #11)
- Hysteroscopy (see Section #15)
- Laparoscopy

Once compiled, this information should be reviewed with the couple, and treatment options should be discussed. Treatment protocols may include:

- Expectant management
- Operative laparoscopy (see Section #27)
- Tubal microsurgery
- Conservative surgery for endometriosis
- Supplemented ovulation induction
- Artificial insemination (see Section #28) via:
  - Split ejaculate
  - Washed sperm intrauterine insemination (WIUI)
- GIFT (see Section #29)
- IVF (see Section #30), with:
  - Laparoscopic egg harvesting OR
  - Transvaginal egg harvesting
- No viable treatment options
- Consideration of adoption

FIGURE 16.1 — **Pelvic Anatomy Assessment at Laparoscopy**

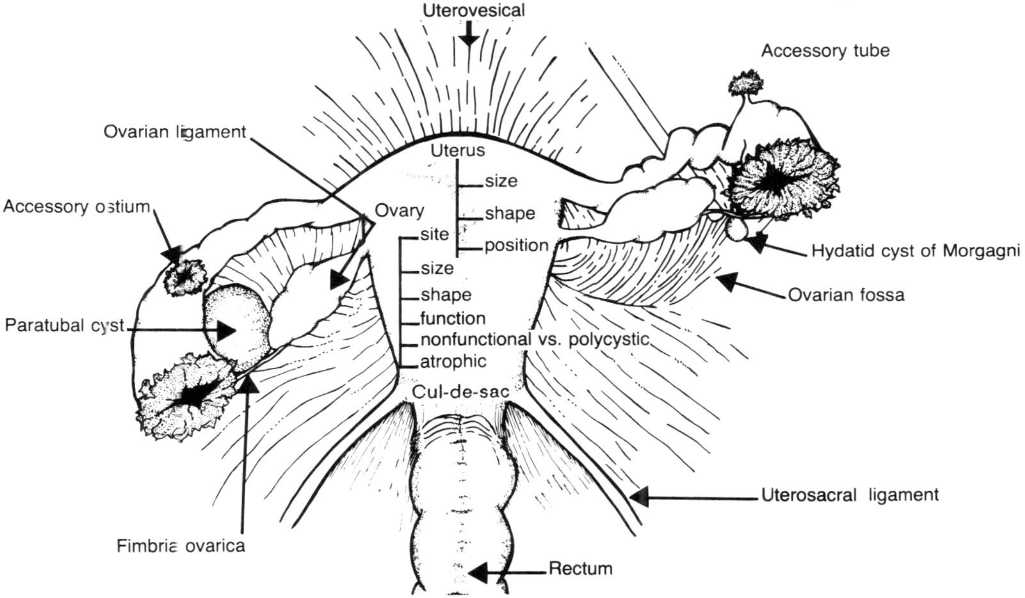

FIGURE 16.2—**Table 1: The American Fertility Society Classification of Adnexal Adhesions**

Patient's Name ______________ Date ________ Chart # ________

Age _____ G ___ P _____ Sp Ab ___ VTP _____ Ectopic ______ Infertile Yes ______ No ______

Other Significant History (ie, surgery, infection, etc.) ______________

HSG ________ Sonography ______ Photography ______ Laparoscopy ________ Laparotomy ________

	ADHESIONS	**< 1/3 Enclosure**	**1/3 - 2/3 Enclosure**	**> 2/3 Enclosure**
OVARY	R Filmy	1	2	4
	Dense	4	8	16
	L Filmy	1	2	4
	Dense	4	8	16
TUBE	R Filmy	1	2	4
	Dense	4*	8*	16
	L Filmy	1	2	4
	Dense	4*	8*	16

*If the fimbriated end of the fallopian tube is completely enclosed, change the point assignment to 16.

Prognostic Classification for Adnexal Adhesions

		LEFT		RIGHT
A.	Minimal	______	0-5	______
B.	Mild	______	6-10	______
C.	Moderate	______	11-20	______
D.	Severe	______	21-32	______

Treatment (Surgical Procedures): ______

______

______

______

______

Prognosis for Conception & Subsequent Viable Infant**

______	Excellent	(> 75%)
______	Good	(50%-75%)
______	Fair	(25%-50%)
______	Poor	(< 25%)

**Physician's judgment based upon adnexa with least amount of pathology.

Recommended Followup Treatment: ______

______

______

Additional Findings: ______

______

______

______

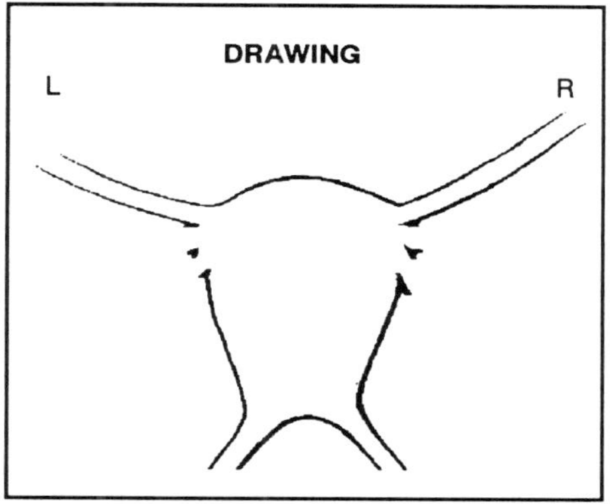

From Buttram VC, et al: Fertil Steril 1988;49:6. Reproduced with permission of the publisher, The American Fertility Society.

FIGURE 16.3 — **The American Fertility Society Revised Classification of Endometriosis**

Patient's Name ______________________ Date __________

Stage I (Minimal) – 1-5
Stage II (Mild) – 6-15
Stage III (Moderate) – 16-40
Stage IV (Severe) – > 40
Total __________

Laparoscopy ______ Laparotomy ______ Photography ______
Recommended Treatment __________

Prognosis __________

		ENDOMETRIOSIS	< 1cm	1-3cm	> 3cm
PERITONEUM		Superficial	1	2	4
		Deep	2	4	6
OVARY	R	Superficial	1	2	4
		Deep	4	16	20
	L	Superficial	1	2	4
		Deep	4	16	20

POSTERIOR CUL-DE-SAC OBLITERATION	**Partial**	**Complete**
	4	40

		ADHESIONS	< 1/3 Enclosure	1/2 - 2/3 Enclosure	> 2/3 Enclosure
OVARY	R	Filmy	1	2	4
		Dense	4	8	16
	L	Filmy	1	2	4
		Dense	4	8	16
TUBE	R	Filmy	1	2	4
		Dense	4*	8*	16
	L	Filmy	1	2	4
		Dense	4*	8*	16

*If the fimbriated end of the fallopian tube is completely enclosed, change the point assignment to 16.

Additional Endometriosis: ______________________

To Be Used with Normal Tubes and Ovaries

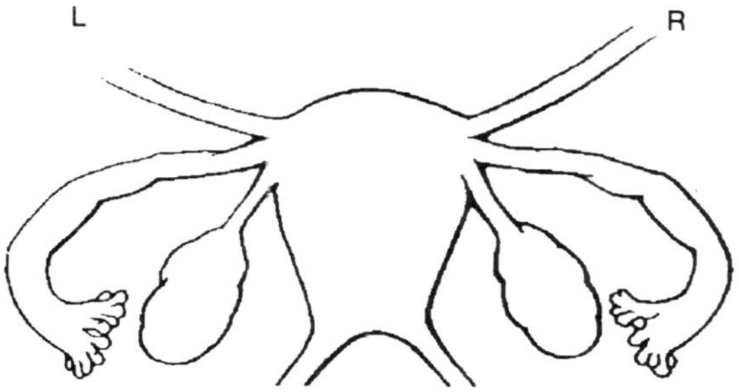

Associated Pathology: ______________________

To Be Used with Abnormal Tubes and/or Ovaries

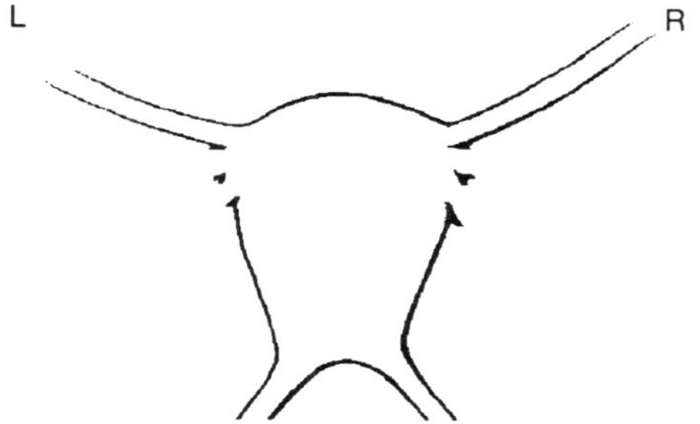

From Andrews WC, et al: Fertil Steril 1985;43:3. Reproduced with permission of the publisher, The American Fertility Society.

FIGURE 16.4—**Common Puncture Sites of Diagnostic and Operative Laparoscopy**

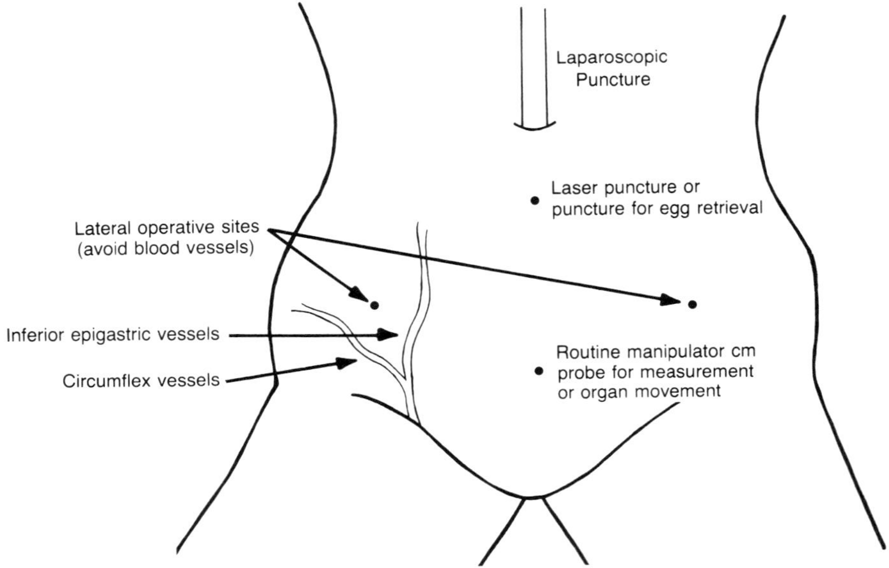

NOTES

#17 Vaginosonography

Definition

Vaginosonography uses high-frequency sound waves emitted by a crystal to record reflections (echoes) from the interfaces of various tissue densities. These reflections are observed as real time ultrasound images. Radiodense and radiolucent variations, dependent on the density of their tissues, allow differentiation of the pelvic organs.

Three different sound frequency probes are available for use in this procedure, including:

- Low frequency (3.5 MHz)—For visualization at depths of 5 to 15 cms but with a loss of detailed resolution
- Intermediate frequency (5 MHz)—For visualization between 2 and 12 cms
- High frequency (6.5 or 7 MHz)—To provide greater resolution and detail; penetration is limited to approximately 1.5 to 7 cms

The introduction of the ultrasound probe into the vagina facilitates a close proximity of the ultrasonic crystal to the target organ (within 3 to 5 cms). This allows the use of higher-frequency probes (5 MHz or 6.5 to 7 MHz) with greater clarity and detailed resolution. The impact of this innovation has been so dramatic that it has revolutionized the practice of infertility care, altering many diagnostic and therapeutic techniques.

The ability to accurately define the size of the ovaries and to observe developing follicles greater than 2 mm in diameter has:

- Provided detail for the close monitoring of ovulation induction
- Facilitated monitoring and ensured the correct timing of HCG injections for multiple ovarian stimulation as required for:
  - IVF
  - GIFT
  - Related procedures

17.

- Provided safe access and control for transvaginal harvesting of ova from the ovaries, reducing the need for a more invasive operative laparoscopic procedure

This close proximity to tissues also precludes the necessity to transfer sound waves via a distended bladder and its associated elevation of the pelvic organs. Additionally, the scan can be completed at the time of pelvic examination for cervical assessment during ovulation induction. Thus, this innovative procedure provides the patient maximal convenience and comfort; she may undergo the procedure with an empty bladder, and she need not make a second visit for ultrasound examination.

The vaginal probe is inserted and a detailed examination of the cervix, uterine cavity, ovaries and oviducts is completed.

Basic Indications

The ease and accuracy with which the vaginosonogram can be performed allows for unproblematic repeat examinations and safe monitoring of ovulation induction, stimulated by HMG, pure FSH or combinations of clomiphene citrate and HMG. Results of ovulation induction, seen at vaginosonogram, will:

- Confirm normal ovarian status and exclude residual cysts before medications for ovulation induction are repeated
- Assess the mid-cycle proliferative phase for both spontaneous and medically-induced ovulation
- Confirm maturity of dominant follicle(s) with a view to possible HCG injection for oocyte retrieval techniques

Clinical Procedure

To perform the vaginosonography, physicians are to:

- Place the patient in the lithotomy position
- Perform a pelvic examination, and document the status of the uterus, ie, antiverted or retroverted

- Complete a cervical examination, assessing and documenting the degree of opening or closing of the os, together with mucus aspiration for assessment and documentation for:
  - Spinnbarkeit
  - Ferning
  - Sperm, via high-power field, for speed of forward progression
- Withdraw the speculum
- Cover the vaginal probe with a sterile, non-spermicidal condom or rubber glove which has been lubricated:
  - Internally with radiolucent jelly
  - Externally with water to avoid the spermicidal effect of the jelly
- Advise the patient of the insertion of the vaginal probe; gently pass the probe into the vagina
- Screen longitudinal and horizontal (sagittal and transverse) sections of the:
  - Cervix
  - Cervical canal
  - Uterine cavity
- Check the uterus and review the endometrial cavity, documenting the endometrium's:
  - Thickness
  - Pattern
- Direct the probe to an adnexa, and follow the fallopian tube to the ovary, defining and measuring its longitudinal and horizontal diameters
- Visualize the fallopian tube, documenting:
  - Ovarian size
  - Presence or absence of follicles (by diameter)
- Measure and document all follicles greater than 5 mm in diameter
- Direct the probe to the opposite adnexa and follow the same protocol as above
- Screen the cul-de-sac for free fluid
- Document findings (a simple method of diagrammatic documentation of follicular findings is illustrated in Figure 17.1), filing the figures one on top

of another, so that, in turning the diagrams over, the number and rate of change in follicular growth is immediately obtained

- Withdraw all instruments
- Immediately document all findings

Results

In classic, "normal," spontaneous ovulation:

- The dominant follicle will mature and rupture at diameters of 18 to 25 mm
- Secondary follicles, noted in the dominant ovary, are usually from 10 to 12 mm in diameter, and a few follicles of less than 10 mm in diameter may be seen in the opposite ovary

When clomiphene citrate is used for ovulation induction, the dominant follicle usually matures to a slightly larger size (22 to 30 mm) prior to rupture. With HMG, the dominant follicle usually ruptures when it reaches 18 to 25 mm. Therefore, it is common practice to induce ovulation with HCG when a mature follicle exhibits these diameters using clomiphene citrate or HMG therapy.

These basic principles are modified in the multiple ovulation induction protocols of "hyperstimulation" used for IVF and GIFT. Under normal conditions, however, HCG is withheld if the threat of ovarian hyperstimulation is indicated by:

- Multiple dominant follicles
- Multiple secondary follicles
- Bilateral multiple follicles
- "Honeycombing" of the ovaries
- A plasma estradiol rate of elevation greater than three-fold within 24 hours

Each laboratory and clinic sets its own safe maximum hyperstimulation levels, usually ranging between 800 and 1,600 pg/mL.

Patients at most risk for hyperstimulation are those with:

- Overt oligomenorrhea
- Amenorrhea
- Polycystic ovarian syndrome

During vaginosonography, follicle rupture can be confirmed once ovulation occurs. The collapse of the follicle can be noted in association with the presence of free fluid in the cul-de-sac. For this examination, the patient is placed in reverse Trendelenburg position or sitting up on her elbows or hands, so that fluid may accumulate in the cul-de-sac.

Persistence of the dominant follicle in the presence of a temperature rise and/or of elevation of progesterone indicates luteinized unruptured follicle (LUF) syndrome. This implies formation of a corpus luteum, yet failure of ovum release from the ovarian surface.

Diagnosis of LUF syndrome is primarily made via ultrasonography. In the past, the diagnosis was by laparoscopic assessment of the ovaries following ovulation, to confirm the presence of luteinized follicles in the absence of an ovarian stigma. Diagnosis implies that luteinization of the granulosa and theca cells of the follicle has occurred but that rupture of the follicle's surface and ovum release has not.

Management of LUF Syndrome

LUF syndrome is managed by:

- Seeking the cause, such as:
  - General endocrinopathy
  - Endometriosis
  - Hyperandrogenism
  - Hyperprolactinemia
  - Parovarian adhesions
- Treating the cause, by:
  - Reducing hyperandrogenism
  - Reducing hyperprolactinemia
  - Pharmacologically or surgically treating endometriosis
  - Surgically removing parovarian adhesions, by:
    - Laparoscopy
    - Laparotomy
- Supplementing ovulation induction, by:
  - Clomiphene citrate plus HCG

- Administering HCG therapy at mid-cycle, the treatment of choice for hormonal causes, such as:
  - General endocrine
  - Inadequate LH surge at mid-cycle (commonly due to endometriosis)
- Treating local causes, such as:
  - Pelvic inflammatory disease (PID)
  - Endometriosis
  - Possible peritubal adhesions
- Resolving local causes, ie, removing physical barriers to the ovarian surfaces, by:
  - Laparoscopic laser or coagulation
  - Microelectrodes or lasers at laparotomy

Early Diagnosis of Pregnancy

Vaginosonography provides a detailed, close view of the adnexa and uterine cavity, thus assisting in early diagnosis of pregnancy. Gestation may be confirmed as a 4- to 5-mm sac at 15 to 18 days after ovulation by this method.

Additionally, this procedure allows assessment of an adnexal mass with greater detail, and the accuracy of diagnosis of ectopic pregnancy is elevated from 60 to 90 percent (approximately) using this method; the operator must be extremely gentle and cautious in using the probe when clinical circumstances suggest a possible tubal gestation.

In assessing early pregnancy, vaginosonography provides great insight and detail of:

- Stages of development of the gestational ring
- The yolk sac
- Presence of a fetal heartbeat

When combined with abdominal ultrasound, the two methods complement each other in achieving a more detailed assessment of early gestational pathology.

Vaginosonography in ART: Basic Principles of Transvaginal Ovum Retrieval

The lucid detail of each follicle, following multiple ovulation induction, may be provided by vaginosonography. This capability facilitates the harvesting of ova via transvaginal ultrasound-guided needle methods. As a result, assisted reproductive techniques (ART) benefit greatly. ART methods include:

- IVF (see Sections #25 and #30)
- GIFT (see Sections #25 and #29)
- ZIFT/TET (see Sections #25 and #30)

Clinical Procedure

See Section #30.

FIGURE 17.1 – **Ultrasound Monitoring of Ovaries – Method of Documentation of Ovarian Response in Ovulation Induction**

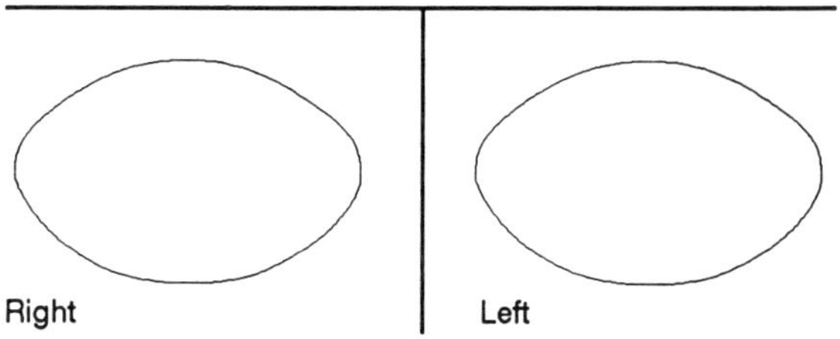

DAY 2 – Basal assessment – No follicular activity.

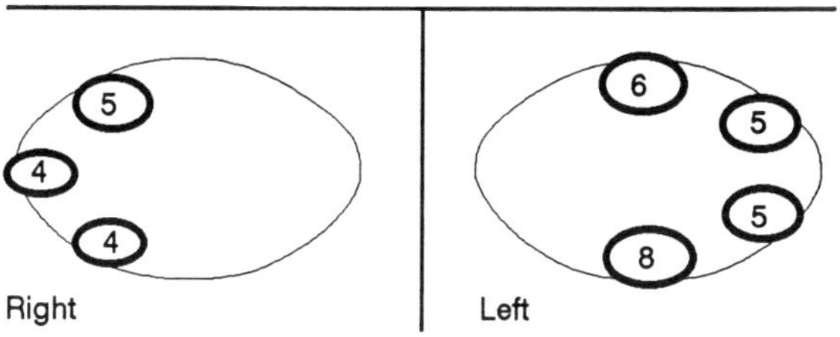

DAY 6 – Early follicular development.

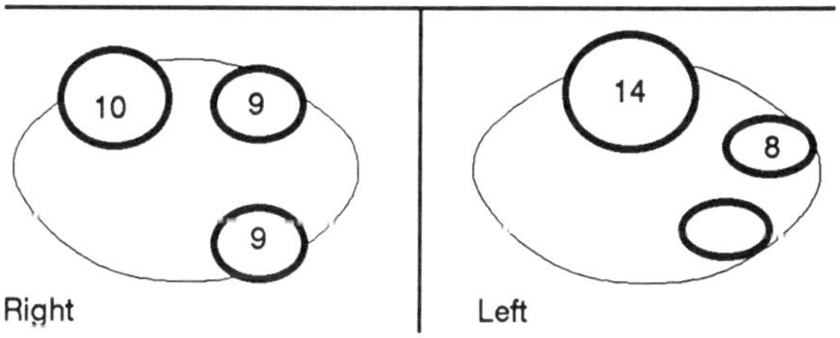

DAY 11 – Follicular growth and establishment of follicular dominance in the left ovary.

NOTE: Numbers depicting follicular development are given in millimeters.

#18 Male Factor

The cause of infertility in 30 to 40 percent of couples is attributable to the male factor, as determined by abnormal:

- Postcoital test (see Section #19)
- Semen analysis (see Section #10)

Assessment of Causes

A detailed history should be made of the causes for infertility relating to the male factor, followed by a complete physical examination (see Section #7).

Infertility may also be due to:

- Sexual dysfunction, including:
  - Impotence, psychological vs. organic, due to:
    - Diabetes mellitus
    - Neurological problems
    - Vascular problems
  - Premature ejaculation
  - Situational orgasmic dysfunction, ie, the ability to attain orgasm at masturbation but not with vaginal penetration
- Immunological causes, ie, the presence of antisperm antibodies to the head, neck and/or tail of sperm, indicated by:
  - IgA
  - IgG
  - IgM

Investigations

The investigations used to determine causes of infertility in the male factor are the same as the basal workups ordered for determining causes of abnormal semen analysis (see Section #10) and negative postcoital tests (see Section #19).

Management

Treatment protocols for infertility relating to the male factor include:

- Sexual counseling

18.

- Assessment of stress factors and changes in lifestyle regarding the use of:
  - Drugs
  - Alcohol
  - Tobacco
- Weight reduction for the obese
- Counseling to wear loose-fitting undergarments
- Counseling to opt for cold thermal activities (eg, swimming) and to avoid heat-related activities (eg, saunas and hot tubs)
- Ligation or balloon occlusion of varicocele
- Testicular biopsy in severe:
  - Oligospermia
  - Azoospermia
- Vasogram and possible exploration of ejaculatory ducts via microsurgical:
  - Vasovasostomy
  - Vasoepididymostomy
  - Transurethral exploration
- Possible hormonal therapy, dependent on test results; therapy may include:
  - Low-dose clomiphene citrate
  - HCG, for low plasma testosterone associated with low levels of LH
  - HMG, for true hypogonadotropic hypogonadism
  - Parlodel®, for hyperprolactinemia exclusive of prolactinoma (seen at CAT scan)
  - Low-dose androgen (eg, testosterone at 5 to 10 mg daily for 40 to 60 days), for selected cases of asthenospermia
  - Thyroid replacement, for proven hypothyroidism
  - Corticosteroids, in selected cases with sperm antibodies
  - ART, including:
    - Sperm enhancement (see Section #28)
    - GIFT (see Section #29)
    - IVF (see Section #30)
    - ZIFT/TET (see Section #30)

In all cases of hormonal therapy, plasma testosterone must be monitored initially, at 10 days and subsequently at three- to six-week intervals. A semen analysis should be performed and assessed every 60 days to ensure a positive response to therapy. If no change or a relative decline in seminal parameters occurs, hormonal therapy should be discontinued immediately.

Hormonal treatment of the male continues to be controversial, and the prognosis has been difficult to predict. Notwithstanding, under urological guidance, selected patients may benefit from these therapies.

In principle, an attempt should be made to supplement the function of the male's normal spermatozoa within the ejaculate and to select healthy, active sperm for such ART methods as:

- Sperm preparation for WIUI (see Section #28)
- Swim up technique and selection (see Section #28)
- Use of pre-incubated (capacitation) sperm for:
  - GIFT (see Section #29)
  - IVF (see Section #30)
  - ZIFT/TET (see Section #30)
- Zona splitting and/or drilling for IVF

NOTES

#19 The Abnormal Postcoital Test: Mucus Factor

Definition

An abnormal postcoital test (PCT) is indicated by the absence or paucity of spermatozoa in the cervical mucus within two to six hours of intercourse.

Causes of Abnormal PCTs

While the most common cause of an abnormal PCT is incorrect timing of the test (especially not completing the test immediately prior to ovulation [see Section #12]), other factors need to be considered.

For the male, causes for abnormal semen analysis (see Section #10) are also causes for the abnormal PCT; these include:

- Azoospermia–The absence of spermatozoa
- Oligospermia–Low numbers of spermatozoa
- Asthenospermia–Poor motility of spermatozoa
- History of mumps
- Neoplasms
- Systemic and hormonal damage
- Presence of antisperm antibodies
- Faulty coital technique or sexual dysfunction (see Section #18)

For the female, abnormal PCTs may be caused by:

- Cervical disorders, including:
  - DES exposure
  - Previous surgery
  - Cryotherapy
  - Cone biopsy
  - Aggressive laser vaporization
  - Cervicitis, acute and chronic, such as:
    - Chlamydia
    - Mycoplasma
    - Ureaplasma
  - Recurrent cervical:
    - Infection
    - Ectropion
    - Erosion

- Carcinoma
- *In situ* carcinoma
- Mucus antisperm antibodies
- Systemic and/or hormonal problems, including:
  - Hypoestrogenism
  - Antiestrogens, via the administration of:
    - Androgens
    - Progestins
    - Clomiphene citrate
  - Hyperprolactinemia

19.

Immunological causes may occur in the male or female. Antisperm antibodies directed at the head, neck or tail of the sperm may be present. These IgA, IgM or IgG antibodies to the sperm may be found:

- In the male's:
  - Serum
  - Spermatozoa
  - Semen
- In the female's:
  - Serum
  - Cervical mucus

Basic Assessment

Causes of abnormal PCT relating to the male are assessed by:

- Semen analysis (see Section #10)
- Noting heat factors, such as:
  - The use of hot tubs and saunas
  - Jogging and excessive athletic exercise
  - Tight, ill-fitting undergarments
  - Working in hot environments
  - Smoking
- Endocrine factors (see Section #13)

Factors affecting the female cervical mucus include:

- Wrong timing of PCT (see Section #12)
- Infections, especially cervical; these should be cultured and treated
- Hypoestrogenic (all endocrine) situations, from the:

- Hypothalamus
- Pituitary
- Gonad
- Adrenal
- Thyroid
- Iatrogenic, both progestins and androgens

Principles of Management

Treatment for the abnormal PCT in the female includes:

- For cervical infections–
  - Topical sulfa creams
  - Systemic ofloxacin/doxycycline/ampicillin therapy
- For chronic cervical erosions–
  - Cauterization
  - Laser vaporization
- To supplement ovulation induction at higher estrogen levels–
  - Clomiphene citrate–Mid-cycle estradiol levels greater than 300 pg/mL and absence of cervical mucus indicates an antiestrogenic effect of the drug

If the abnormal PCT results from clomiphene citrate use, the regimen may be supplemented with estrogens and, possibly, guaifenesins. If supplemented estrogen and guaifenesins evoke no response, HMG therapy may be considered.

If all other parameters are normal and the absence of cervical mucus is related to previous cryotherapy, DES exposure or cervical stenosis or excision, the cervix may be bypassed and washed sperm intrauterine inseminaton (WIUI) attempted (see Section #28). WIUI is commonly completed in association with supplemented ovulation induction, including clomiphene citrate plus HCG or HMG therapy (if the clomiphene citrate is not successful). Progesterone supplementation of the luteal phase may also be indicated (see Section #20).

NOTES

#20 Ovulatory Disorders

Clinical Presentation

Patients with ovulatory disorders may present with histories including any of the following:

- Amenorrhea
- Regular menstrual cycles with mild or minimal premenstrual symptoms
- Absence of symptoms
- Mid-cycle pain
- Dysmenorrhea
- Cycle variations:
  - Short follicular/proliferative phase
  - Long follicular/proliferative phase
  - Slow thermal shift
  - Short secretory/luteal phase
  - Minimal thermal shift during secretory/luteal phase
  - Stepladder rise in thermal shift

Any of these symptoms may be associated with:

- General stress
- Major weight gain or loss
- Athletic pursuits, strenuous exercise
- Galactorrhea
- Hirsutism
- Previous sterilization
- Endometriosis
- Premenstrual and/or postmenstrual spotting
- Mid-cycle bleeding as a consistent pattern

The temperature graph may reveal a menstrual cycle that exhibits:

- No change
- Uniphasia, consistent with amenorrhea
- Various graph abnormalities, consistent with regular menses but demonstrating ovulatory dysfunction (see *Cycle variations* above)

Examination

The physical examination will reveal:

- Obesity or thinness
- Hirsutism

- Virilism
- Hair distribution
- Galactorrhea
- Low body fat percentile
- Anorexic disposition
- Dental damage (possibly from bulimia)
- Cushingoid facies
- Buffalo hump
- Acanthosis nigricans
- Vaginal dryness and/or absence of cervical mucus in hypoestrogenic patients
- Excessive cervical mucus secretions in "estrus" pattern (classically with oligomenorrhea; it is indicative of increased estrogen activity with the absence of progesterone and anovulation)
- A small uterus in hypoestrogenic women
- A bulky uterus in hyperestrogenic women
- Palpable polycystic ovaries

20.

Investigations

The investigation of ovulatory disorders begins with a detailed history, physical examination and laboratory assessment, noting:

- Cervical mucus with clear spinnbarkeit ferning (estrogenic)
- Plasma progesterone
  - Less than 2 ng/mL indicates anovulation
  - Three to 15 ng/mL indicates ovulation with possible secretory/luteal phase deficiency
  - Greater than 15 ng/mL indicates adequate secretory/luteal phase
- Levels of:
  - TSH
  - Prolactin
  - DHEAS
  - Testosterone
  - Free testosterone
  - 17-hydroxyprogesterone (if indicated)

  Plasma androgens and prolactin should be drawn during the follicular/proliferative phase of the menstrual cycle at least two hours postprandial and prior to examination of the patient

- Elevated cortisol, tested by overnight dexamethasone suppression (1 mg is taken at 11:00 p.m. on the prior evening, repeating DHEAS levels at 8:00 a.m. Cushing's syndrome is excluded if results are less than 5 ng/dL)
- Pelvic ultrasound:
  - A small uterus, which is relatively quiescent, and barely visible ovaries indicate hypoestrogenic situations
  - A normal size uterus and polycystic ovaries indicate polycystic ovarian syndrome
- Pituitary CAT scan and/or nuclear magnetic resonance imaging (MRI) should be performed for patients presenting with:
  - Hyperprolactinemia
  - Cushing's syndrome
  - Hypogonadotropic hypogonadism
- Adrenal and ovarian CAT scan and/or MRI scan is performed in cases of non-suppressible adrenal and/or ovarian hyperandrogenism. Selective venous catheterization may be indicated if elevated plasma androgens are present and the source (adrenal or ovarian) is difficult to ascertain
- Progesterone challenge test differentiates estrogenic and hypoestrogenic patients. Because progesterone or progestins only act on estrogen-primed receptors and target tissues, the absence of basal estrogen activity does not facilitate bleeding after progesterone administration:
  - If the patient demonstrates vaginal withdrawal bleeding following administration of progestins. A basal estrogen-primed endometrium that will respond to ovulation induction with clomiphene citrate is indicated
  - If no bleeding occurs. The patient is hypoestrogenic and will require hypothalamic-pituitary stimulation or replacement agents (ie, HMG or GnRH therapy). Premature menopause should be excluded before beginning therapy

A negative pregnancy test should be confirmed prior to performing progesterone challenge test. For the test, patients are given:

- Usually, daily MPA 10 mg orally for five days (twice daily for obese patients) OR
- Progesterone in oil 100 to 200 mg IM (200 mg for women weighing 150 lbs. or more; the dose is weight-dependent)

Bleeding should occur within three to five days of discontinuing MPA or approximately 14 days after the initial dose.

CAVEAT: In a small percentage of patients, progesterone induces an LH surge, ovulation occurs and the anticipated menses occurs approximately 14 days later.

Principles of Management

Ovulation Induction

After causes of anovulation are assessed and a diagnosis is established, therapy for ovulation induction is begun, unless the diagnosis indicates other specific therapies. Ovulation may be induced by the use of:

- Clomiphene citrate
- Clomiphene citrate and HCG
- Bromocriptine
- Corticosteroids
- Estrogen/progestin combinations
- HMG
- GnRH
- GnRH agonists

CLOMIPHENE CITRATE

Clomiphene citrate, a derivative of the primitive estrogen Tace®, functions primarily as a hypothalamic-pituitary stimulant because of its antiestrogenic properties.

The administration of clomiphene citrate results in depletion of estrogens from hypothalamic-pituitary receptors, with resultant stimulation of gonadotropins, primarily FSH production. Such stimulation initiates follicular maturation and a cascade of estrogen production, with subsequent further stimulation of FSH, which builds up estrogen and FSH receptors in the granulosa cells of the primordial follicle. The resultant estradiol surge initiates an LH surge which triggers ovulation (see Sections #2 through #5).

Clomiphene citrate 50 mg is administered on days five through nine of the menstrual cycle in the totally anovulatory patient and on days three through seven in the dysovulatory patient. The initial antiestrogenic response may be accompanied by:

- Vaginal dryness
- Hot flashes
- Nausea
- Dizziness
- Occasional visual disturbances (if these are significant, the drug is discontinued)

Ovulation most commonly occurs seven to 10 days after the last clomiphene citrate pill is administered; thus, most patients ovulate during days 17 through 20. Coitus should be timed accordingly.

In menstruating women with inadequate ovulation and/or secretory/luteal phase deficiency, the clomiphene citrate should be administered early in the menstrual cycle to coincide with early FSH stimulation (approximately the third day of menses). Pregnancy should first be excluded in these cases.

Positive effects are indicated by:

- Elevation of plasma estrogen with improvement in cervical mucus
- Adequate preparation of the dominant follicle by enrichment of FSH and E_2 receptors
- Adequate enrichment of the endometrium with estrogen and progesterone receptors, facilitating a positive response to progesterone
- Enhancement of the LH surge and subsequent adequate output of progesterone by the adequately-prepared and stimulated corpus luteum

- Elevated progesterone levels on adequately-prepared endometrial receptors (such elevation enhances the adequacy of the endometrium during the secretory/luteal phase)

The potential negative effects of this therapy include:

- Antiestrogenic response, with absence and/or thickening of the cervical mucus
- Variable LH response
- Antiestrogenic effects on the endometrium, with 20 to 30 percent incidence of luteal phase deficiency and discrepancy in dated endometrial biopsy. This must be excluded, particularly when observing clomiphene-enhanced, "normal" progesterone values. For example, a progesterone level of 17 to 20 ng/mL may be associated with a major lag in endometrial response, as assessed on endometrial biopsy
- The occurrence of ovarian cysts, primarily because of failure of stimulated follicles to rupture
- Hyperstimulation syndrome

Negative responses are most common in thin, low body weight patients and those in whom clomiphene citrate is used repetitively, because its slow metabolism (10 to 17 days) may result in cumulative effects. Because of the drug's dose/weight relationship, the dosage for patients weighing less than 105 lbs. should be halved.

Recommended Doses and Monitoring

Prior to clomiphine citrate administration, a pelvic exam should be performed to confirm the absence of ovarian masses or cysts. If doubt exists, a sonogram should be performed as a baseline study.The initial dose (one-half to one tablet, ie, 25 to 50 mg) is administered for five days, beginning on cycle day three to five. Approximately seven to 10 days after the regimen is completed, patients should be given:

- Postcoital test
- Vaginal sonography to confirm the number and diameter of follicles stimulated (if more than two

follicles are stimulated to more than 20 mms, HCG should not be administered)

- Cervical mucus check
- Sperm penetration of mucus test (if intercourse has occurred)
- HCG 5,000 IU, if two follicles or less are present with diameters greater than 20 mm and previous progesterone has been inadequate (ie, less than 10 ng/mL)

Plasma progesterone is documented approximately seven days after the HCG injection (if given). The endometrial biopsy must be performed within three months of the commencement of clomiphene citrate therapy in order to exclude an iatrogenic luteal phase deficiency, a condition which occurs in 20 to 30 percent of cases.

If secretory/luteal phase deficiency is confirmed in a second premenstrual endometrial biopsy, progesterone vaginal suppositories 25 mg twice daily should be given after ovulation. Subsequent endometrial biopsy should confirm correction of the defect with "in-phase" endometrium.

Some clinicians advise increasing the amount of clomiphene citrate when secretory/luteal phase deficiency is noted. This protocol should be directed at the patient whose initial ovulatory response has been totally inadequate (ie, with plasma progesterone levels of 7 to 10 ng/mL). If progesterone values are 17 to 25 ng, increasing the clomiphene citrate may:

- Over stimulate the patient
- Aggravate the secretory/luteal phase deficiency observed on endometrial biopsy, especially in patients having negative mucus "antiestrogenic" responses to clomiphene citrate which may be further aggravated by the increased dosage

In some patients, the secretory/luteal phase deficit cannot be corrected, despite positive responses of:

- Adequate estradiol rise
- Normal cervical mucus
    - Plasma progesterone above 15 ng/mL
    - Supplemented by progesterone suppositories

This situation is rare, but most of these patients respond to HMG therapy. It is possible that use of gonadotropins excludes the antiestrogenic effects of the clomiphene citrate, but no hard evidence exists to confirm this speculation.

Negative Cervical Mucus

It is essential that the cervical mucus of patients on clomiphene citrate be assessed at the correct time during the menstrual cycle. Timing is confirmed by one of the following:

- LH surge via surge guide monitoring
- Estradiol surge
- Adequate maturation of ovarian follicles via ultrasound

After confirmation, a plasma estradiol should be drawn if the patient exhibits no cervical mucus or cervical mucus that is thickened or cellular.

If estradiol levels are assessed to be less than 200 pg/mL, the patient has probably been given an inadequate amount of clomiphene citrate and the dosage should be increased.

If plasma estradiol is greater than 250 pg/mL, the antiestrogenic effect of the clomiphene citrate likely is dominant. This may be corrected with guaifenesin given on cycle days nine through 13 or with supplemental estrogens (eg, ethinyl estradiol) given daily from approximately cycle day nine in increasing and then decreasing increments of 0.2, 0.2, 0.4, 0.4, 0.6, 0.6, 0.4 and 0.2 μg.

Failure of these methods to improve the cervical mucus indicates the need for HMG therapy. Careful and timely administration of HMG after repeated negative cervical mucus in patients given clomiphene citrate facilitates estradiol production with no antiestrogenic effects.

Women on clomiphene citrate whose estradiol levels are above 1,000 pg/mL and who still have no cervical mucus have been observed, after HMG therapy, to have plasma estradiol levels of 250 to 300 pg/mL and perfect, abundant, clear, cervical mucus. When HMG is used to correct the mucus factor in such patients, it should not be necessary to elevate the plasma estradiol above 500 pg/mL. Hyperstimulation of the patient is not the intended goal in these cases, as it is in the preparation for egg harvesting for procedures such as IVF and GIFT.

CAVEAT: HMG should only be administered by those trained and thoroughly experienced in its potential side effects and serious hyperstimulation complications.

CLOMIPHENE CITRATE AND HCG

Clomiphene citrate therapy alone, administered incrementally in dosages of 25 to 200 mg per day, should be tried before adding human chorionic gonadotropin (HCG) to the regimen. Clomiphene may be tried in very obese women in dosages of up to 200 mg per day, since a dose/weight relationship exists for this drug.

Dosages for thin women (ie, those weighing less than 115 lbs.) should not exceed 150 mg per day. Larger doses in low body weight patients are most commonly associated with negative antiestrogenic effects of clomiphene citrate, including:

- Absence of cervical mucus
- Secretory/luteal phase deficiency

The risk of hyperstimulation in thin women is also significant.

The incremental increases in clomiphene citrate should be carefully monitored, observing its effects on the patient. If ovulation occurs with one or two mature follicles, yet the thermal shift with the plasma progesterone is slow (in the range of 5 to 10 ng/mL), most likely, the only deficit is an inadequate LH surge. Such patients will benefit from HCG, 5,000 IU IM given at mid-cycle, which is timed by monitoring the estradiol levels and measuring dominant follicles by ultrasound.

If an inadequate LH surge is the only deficit in these patients, the need for large doses of clomiphene citrate should be reviewed, and timely administration of HCG would be preferred. If ovulation can only be accomplished with high doses of clomiphene citrate, the cumulative antiestrogen problems (absence of mucus and secretory/luteal phase deficient endometrium) are avoided by proceeding to HMG therapy.

High miscarriage rates in patients taking large doses of clomiphene citrate without HCG supplements are probably a result of the antiestrogenic effects of clomiphene citrate and the coincidental inadequate LH surge. Hypothetically, an adequate LH surge should result in an adequate output of progesterone from the corpus luteum in these women.

The dosage of clomiphene citrate should be carefully monitored so that only the minimum dose necessary to achieve adequate follicular maturation and ovulation is given. Timely administration of HCG supplements this activity.

To achieve positive results (ie, adequate ovulation, adequate plasma progesterone and normal luteal phase [confirmed at endometrial biopsy]), it is always preferable to administer a lesser amount of clomiphene citrate (eg, 75 mg) for five days with HCG 5,000 IU at mid-cycle than to give clomiphene citrate in daily high dosages (200 to 250 mg). Given the drug's inherent antiestrogenic effects, it is unlikely that large doses will result in normal physiological ovulation, particularly in low body weight patients.

CAVEAT: HCG should never be administered blindly. To avoid risks and complications of hyperstimulation, the status of patients (ie, the number of mature follicles present and/or estradiol levels) should always be determined by pelvic ultrasound (see Section #17) prior to HCG administration, regardless of clomiphene citrate and/or HMG use.

BROMOCRIPTINE

Bromocriptine is a dopamine agonist which lowers prolactin secretion. Patients presenting with hyperprolactinemia (ie, levels greater than 25 ng/mL) or with hypoestrogenism and upper to normal prolactin levels are evaluated via CAT scan or MRI pituitary scan, when indicated, to exclude pituitary adenoma before bromocriptine is administered.

The initial therapy is bromocriptine alone, since its administration normalizes ovulation in most patients with elevated prolactin levels. If there is failure of adequate ovulation despite correcting the prolactin level, further stimulation with clomiphene citrate and, if necessary, HMG should be considered, though such combined therapy may result in major hyperstimulation.

Prolactin levels should always be normalized before other agents are added to the bromocriptine therapy, and negative effects of prolactin on estrogen and progesterone receptors must be corrected before stimulation by additional agents is attempted. Side effects of bromocriptine include:

- Nasal stuffiness
- Nausea
- Mild gastrointestinal disturbances
- Postural hypotension

Patients should be counseled regarding these possible side effects, which may be prevented if the drug is taken at bedtime in doses of 1.25 mg for the first three days and in standard doses of 2.5 mg thereafter.

During therapy, patients are also advised to:

- Drink abundant amounts of fluids
- Rise slowly from sitting or prone positions
- Avoid taking hot showers

Occasionally, it will also be necessary for patients to supplement their diets with additional salt and/or caffeinated drinks until adequate doses of bromocriptine can be established without the side effects of postural hypotension.

The effects of the bromocriptine dosage on plasma prolactin should be checked at seven- to 10-day intervals and the dosage adjusted until normal prolactin levels are established.

If ovulation is inadequate despite correction of prolactin levels, clomiphene citrate may be administered, beginning with the lowest dose (dependent on body weight) of 25 or 50 mg per day for five days. Subsequent monitoring and decisions about HCG and/or supplementation with progesterone are then assessed (see above).

NOTE: Bromocriptine should be discontinued five days before any surgical procedure to prevent drug interactions related to vascular lability.

CORTICOSTEROIDS

Patients who have achieved ovulation induction with clomiphene citrate yet have elevated adrenal androgens (eg, DHEAS greater than 2 ng/dL) should be given dexamethasone in minimum doses to avoid potential harmful side effects of this corticosteroid therapy.

Dexamethasone is administered on days two through 16 of the menstrual cycle if DHEAS is mildly elevated. If DHEAS is above 4 to 6 ng/dL, patients should be given an initial dexamethasone suppression test to rule out possible adrenal tumor. Once adrenal tumor is excluded, dexamethasone may be administered continuously and discontinued once pregnancy is confirmed.

To avoid gastrointestinal ulceration, patients should take dexamethasone at bedtime with food. Physicians should counsel patients to be aware that this is corticosteroid therapy and that, even at low dosages, refractoriness of adrenal response can occur in circumstances of major stress.

This therapy has resulted in a higher incidence of ovulation and pregnancy than clomiphene citrate alone in patients with adrenal hyperandrogenism.

ESTROGEN/PROGESTIN COMBINATIONS
PRIOR TO OVULATION INDUCTION

Patients presenting with markedly elevated androgen (testosterone, androstenedione and DHEAS) levels may be helped by estrogen/progestin combination therapy (birth control pills [OCs]). This lowering of androgens prior to ovulation induction may:

- Facilitate ovulation adequacy
- Exclude the presence of an autonomous testosterone secretory tumor
- Be associated with a lower incidence of miscarriage

This hormonal maneuver should also be considered for patients with markedly elevated androgen levels (particularly, those who have previously conceived and miscarried) who also have inadequate ovulation despite treatment with:

- Clomiphene citrate
- Parlodel®
- Dexamethasone

HMG

NOTE: This manual does not document protocols for the use of HMG and/or associated purified FSH for hyperstimulation in follicular recruitment of harvested oocytes for use in the GIFT, IVF, ZIFT and TET procedures. Such protocols are applicable only in specialized IVF centers. Recommendations in this text are confined to normal ovulation induction with HMG for the purpose of achieving a single pregnancy. Understanding the difference in these two situations is critical to the use of these agents.

Patients presenting with anovulation or ovulatory dysfunction may be refractory to the above simplified modalities of treatment. Human menopausal gonadotropins (HMG) may be given to these patients and to those who are:

- Hypoestrogenic and experience no vaginal bleeding with a plasma progesterone test
- Hypogonadotropic, showing:
  - Low FSH and LH associated with hypothalamic amenorrhea
  - Variations of normal gonadotropin levels but abnormal menstrual patterns

HMG is usually administered as combinations of FSH and LH 75 mL IU/ampule (Pergonal®) or as pure FSH 75 IU (Metrodin®). HMG directly stimulates the ovaries, and, although ovarian response is unpredictable, such response is generally proportional to the amount of gonadotropin stimulation in a particular cycle. Every patient's response is different. Additionally, patients' individual cycles may differ from one month to the next. Patients should be closely monitored and meticulously supervised; the likelihood of hyperstimulation is reduced when individualized and disciplined treatment protocols are maintained.

After a patient is diagnosed as having hypogonadotropic hypogonadism, exhibiting no vaginal bleeding with plasma progesterone test or failing to conceive with other methods of ovulation induction, the couple is counseled regarding the:

- Administration of HMG injections between 3:00 and 7:00 p.m. (ideally, the husband is taught to administer the injections)
- Need for continued monitoring, including:
  - Repeat visits for pelvic ultrasound
  - Estradiol measurements every other day, unless otherwise indicated (measurements may need to be taken daily)
- Possibility of the treatment cycle not being completed due to potential hyperstimulation syndrome (HCG will not be given in this case)
- Need for physical rest and adequate fluid intake during the postovulatory stage when variations of hyperstimulation are frequent (ie, days five to 15 *post-administration* of HCG); maintaining a positive fluid intake prevents hemoconcentration or hypovolemia, which can trigger more serious complications

Pergonal® is begun on the second or third day of menses, after a baseline ultrasound confirms the absence of ovarian cysts. One ampule is administered for three days, at which time an ultrasound and plasma estradiol level are repeated; these parameters are checked on alternate days thereafter.

Depending on the response, Pergonal® is increased by one ampule every two to three days. Ideally, a 50-percent incremental rise in blood estradiol levels (to a range of 400 to 800 pg/mL) will occur every day from approximately day seven or eight of stimulation. This is associated with the occurrence or dominance of one or two follicles.

HCG 5,000 IU is administered at mid-cycle if:

- One to two follicles are dominant and greater than 16 mm in diameter

- Multiple secondary or tertiary follicles are absent
- Estradiol is between 400 to 800 pg/mL

Conversely, HCG is withheld if:

- The incremental rise in estradiol has been more than 100 percent per 24 hours
- Multiple primary and secondary follicles are present
- Estradiol is above 1,000 pg/mL

On occasion, it is evident on day eight or nine that no follicle will dominate. If multiple follicles have been stimulated and estradiol levels are elevated far above physiological norms (eg, 1,000 pg/mL [ideal for IVF]) but no follicle dominates, the treatment cycle is aborted at this early stage.

Progesterone vaginal suppositories 25 mg twice daily are administered as routine in patients undergoing HMG therapy, since this may be a significant factor in reducing the high early miscarriage rate seen with HMG therapy.

CAVEAT: HMG (Pergonal®) therapy should be carried out by physicians who have been trained to use this agent. The potential life-threatening risks of severe ovarian hyperstimulation include:

- Major arterial or venous thrombosis
- Massive ascites
- Hydrothorax
- Significant electrolyte disturbances

The use of pure FSH (Metrodin®) has been reserved primarily for patients with polycystic ovarian disease (PCO) and with confirmed elevated LH:FSH ratios or for HMG protocols which attempt to achieve multiple follicular recruitment for egg harvesting for IVF.

Ovarian Hyperstimulation Syndrome

Patients presenting with mild ovarian hyperstimulation syndrome (ie, ovarian enlargement with minimal fluid in the pelvis and a hematocrit below 45 percent) are:

- Confined to bed at home
- Advised to drink abundant fluids

- Advised to monitor urine output
- Measured repeatedly at 48-hour intervals for:
  - Hematocrit
  - Body weight

It is reassuring in almost all patients when:

- Hematocrit stabilizes between 38 and 42 percent
- Adequate urine output is maintained
- Weight gain is less than 5 lbs. from the weight at the time of ovulation

Approximately seven to 10 days after diagnosis, patients will settle, pain is relieved and diuresis occurs. If conception occurs, HCG is discontinued, since further HCG stimulation of the ovaries may cause a deterioration in the patient's condition, occasionally necessitating hospitalization.

Patients with a hematocrit greater than 45 percent in the presence of marked ovarian enlargement (greater than 10 cm) and associated with free fluid in the abdomen or chest are:

- Hospitalized and documented for:
  - Baseline weight
  - CBC
  - SMAC
  - Urine output
- Positioned with the head slightly elevated
- Cautiously administered IV fluids (previous 24-hour output plus 400 mL per 24 hours)
- Monitored twice daily for hematocrit and electrolyte levels

If true hypoalbuminemia is observed, albumin IV may be administered to assist in maintaining fluid within the intravascular compartment.

Tho major deficit in this case is a shift of fluid into the third space and/or pleural cavity, with marked intravascular hemoconcentration and possible decreased renal perfusion. Such hemoconcentration is responsible for the life-threatening complications of disseminated intravascular coagulation (DIC), arterial thrombosis and/or cardiac or cerebral ischemia together with pulmonary and renal shutdown. The major aim of therapy is to carefully increase the intravascular space and achieve adequate tissue perfusion, including renal perfusion and adequate urine output.

At approximately seven to 10 days, the patient will diurese with marked improvement in overall condition. Pregnancy may cause deterioration in the patient's condition. Occasionally, thoracic or pelvic paracentesis may be necessary.

Chronic ascites is rarely a major medical emergency, but in ovarian hyperstimulation, the acute shift of fluid into the abdomen with intravascular changes and hemoconcentration is the major potentially life-threatening problem.

Abdominal palpation should be extremely gentle, and pelvic exam and intercourse are to be avoided to prevent hemorrhage, torsion and/or rupture of the ovary. These complications may necessitate surgery on their own merits; though, fortunately, these disastrous consequences are rare because of physician awareness regarding prevention of potentially serious side effects of therapeutic agents.

GONADOTROPIN RELEASING HORMONE (GnRH)

The use of pulsatile GnRH at pulsed intervals of 90 minutes in patients with an intact hypothalamic-pituitary mechanism will result in pituitary stimulation of the ovary by initiating the release of gonadotropins. Most patients ovulate within 10 to 20 days of administration.

Gonadorelin hydrochloride (Factrel®) is the only commercially-available agent for GnRH pulsed stimulation, though it does not yet have FDA approval for the purpose of ovulation induction. It is primarily indicated for those presenting with hypothalamic amenorrhea and in those with PCO who have had previous hyperstimulation, though, to date, such use has been limited. Although the theoretical risk of hyperstimulation is minimized, hyperstimulation has been documented with this agent, particularly in women with PCO.

GnRH patients carry a portable, computerized, pulsatile pump. Dosages are proportional according to administration by IV or subcutaneous injection. IV administration is pulsed at 25 to 100 ng/kg, whereas subcutaneous doses are 10 to 20 mg/pulse.

Once ovulation has occurred, HCG may be given IM 2,500 IU every three to four days or progesterone vaginal suppositories 25 mg twice daily to support the secretory/luteal phase. Patients taking higher dosages should be monitored with ultrasound every other day to note hyperstimulation and/or multiple births.

CAVEAT: This technique should be used only by those adequately trained in GnRH pulsatile pump therapy.

GnRH AGONIST

GnRH agonist (Lupron® administered as an injection 0.5 to 1 mg daily, or Synarel® 400μ/day intranasally) causes an initial release of gonadotropins and a temporary rise in estradiol, followed by down regulation of the pituitary and a resultant hypogonadotropic, hypoestrogenic state. Although these agents are commonly used to prevent premature LH surges and to synchronize the timing of multiple follicular recruitment for ovum harvesting for IVF and/or GIFT procedures, they also have certain indications to assist supplemented ovulation induction under normal conditions.

Indications for GnRH agonist therapy during ovulation induction include:

- Persistent premature LH surge (repeated on ovulation days seven to 10)
- PCO showing recurrent hyperstimulation

GnRH agonist is administered during the secretory/luteal phase of the pre-treatment cycle or prior to initiating a new cycle. Once estradiol levels are consistently less than 20 pg/mL, HMG therapy is commenced. Larger doses of HMG (eg, two to three ampules a day compared to one per day) should be anticipated.

Intensive monitoring is maintained with ultrasound and estradiol levels performed on alternate days until estradiol surges, after which measurements are taken daily.

CAVEAT: The same precautions are maintained for GnRH agonist therapy as for HMG use (see above). Patients must be informed about the possibility that GnRH antibodies may form and that subsequent menstrual irregularity or ovulatory dysfunction can occur. Although current data suggest that this phenomenon is rare, GnRH agonist therapy has not yet been FDA-approved for ovulation induction. Physicians should obtain patient consent for this therapy.

NOTES

#21 Mechanical Disorders: Uterine

Introduction

Abnormalities of the uterus are a rare cause of infertility and are more commonly related to:

- Recurrent early miscarriage
- Premature delivery

Congenital uterine abnormalities include multiple variations of uteri, including:

- T-shaped, commonly caused by diethylstilbestrol (DES) exposure
- Anvil-shaped
- Septate
- Unicornuate
- Bicornuate
- Uterus didelphys

Patients with congenital fundal anomalies may have associated cervical incompetence and/or secretory/luteal phase defects.

Other uterine abnormalities include:

- Intrauterine synechiae (Asherman's syndrome), most commonly following:
  - Septic postabortal or puerperal curettage
  - Uterine sepsis with associated contraceptive intrauterine device (IUD)
  - Chronic infections, such as tuberculosis (uncommon in the U.S.)
- Submucous fibroids
- Intrauterine polyps or adenomyosis

Clinical Presentation

Patients presenting with uterine abnormalities usually present with:

- Secretory/luteal phase defects
- Recurrent early abortion
- Recurrent premature delivery
- Cervical incompetence
- Third-stage complications, including:
  - Postpartum hemorrhage
  - Retained placenta

Diagnosis

Hysterosalpingography or hysteroscopy will reveal obliteration or distortion of the uterine cavity.

Management

Intrauterine synechiae, intrauterine congenital anomalies, septal defects and polyps are transected and/or removed at hysteroscopy, with laparoscopic monitoring.

If the YAG or KTP-532 laser or operating scissors is used, the uterus is distended (see Section #15) with solutions such as:

- Ringer's lactate
- Sorbitol
- Dextran 70

If electrocoagulation and/or the resectoscope are used, the solution should not contain electrolytes; instead, non-conducting solutions are preferred, such as:

- Five- or 10-percent dextrose
- Sorbitol
- Dextran 70

The adhesions are transected and/or congenital anomalies divided, using operating scissors, KTP-532 or YAG fiberoptic lasers or the resectoscope. Perforation, if it occurs, will be seen laparoscopically. If bleeding is not active, no further procedure is necessary, though coagulation of the bleeding surface will occasionally be required. Rarely, laparotomy is performed to facilitate uterine hemostasis and repair.

Postoperative Management

In most cases, no device or catheter is placed in the uterus after surgery. If extensive lysis of adhesions has been performed, a pediatric Foley's catheter is placed and left in the uterine cavity for two to three days.

All patients are given perioperative antibiotics (eg, third-generation cephalosporin 1 g preoperatively and doxycycline or tetracycline for five to seven days postoperatively).

Conjugated estrogens 1.25 mg twice daily to 2.5 mg four times daily for 40 to 60 days promote regrowth of the endometrium in sites previously occupied by fibrous tissue. During the last five days, MPA 10 mg is given daily to prevent a major bleed. When discontinuing the hormonal therapy, short-term progestin therapy is given. A single course of estrogen should not pose a risk of uterine carcinoma, though excessive progestin administration may undo the potential positive effects of estrogen stimulation.

After this 40- to 60-day period of hormonal therapy, the patient is allowed to menstruate spontaneously. Routine expectant management and/or supplemented ovulation induction is then instituted.

Exclusion of a secretory/luteal phase defect by endometrial biopsy will be necessary in many patients. For patients in early pregnancy, many clinicians give progesterone suppositories 25 mg twice daily until the fetal heart is heard. Others administer progesterone caproate 250 mg once to twice weekly for 12 to 14 weeks or until fetal viability is confirmed at 34 weeks. In some institutions, HCG 2,500 IU to 5,000 IU is given three times per week in an effort to secure trophoblastic development in the relatively inadequate endometrial cavity.

Adenomyosis is managed by danazol (Danocrine®) or GnRH agonist therapy in an effort to shrink the uterus and active abnormal endometrium prior to conception attempts with ovulation induction. The secretory/luteal phase is supported with progesterone therapy.

Association with Cervical Incompetence

Cervical incompetence has been noted in some patients presenting with fundal uterine anomalies. A hysterosalpingogram is performed to check for any funneling or widening of the cervical canal. Prospectively, the canal is examined to assess its state of dilatation.

In early pregnancy, the uterine cavity is monitored by detailed ultrasound and digital assessment. If dilatation is present, cervical cerclage (McDonald suture) is completed to prevent miscarriage or premature delivery.

NOTES

#22 Mechanical Disorders: Tuboperitoneal

Introduction

Tuboperitoneal disorders are intrapelvic mechanical derangements that affect the relationship between the tubes and the ovaries.

Adhesions may result in displacement of the distal end of the oviduct and/or traverse the intervening space between the tube and ovary. The tube may have variations of occlusions, including:

- Partial distal occlusion
- Peritubal adhesions
- Intratubal adhesions
- Phimosis
- Total occlusion with small hydrosalpinges
- Total occlusion with large hydrosalpinges and damaged endo- and myosalpinx

Tubal occlusion commonly occurs at the distal end of the oviduct, less frequently at the proximal isthmus or cornu and rarely at mid-oviduct.

Tuboperitoneal disorders include those associated with endometriosis (see Section #23).

Clinical Presentation and Associations

Tuboperitoneal disorders are associated with:

- DES exposure and congenital tubal anomalies
- Tubal sterilization
- Pelvic infection (eg, gonococcus or chlamydia)
- Pelvic surgery
- Ovarian cystectomy
- Ovarian wedge resection and/or appendectomy associated with ovarian surgery
- Appendectomy and/or drainage of pelvic abscess
- Previous caesarean section
- Intrapelvic surgery including myomectomy
- Postpartum or postabortal sepsis
- Previous contraceptive intrauterine device (IUD)

Diagnosis

Hysterosalpingogram and/or laparoscopy is performed after ensuring that patients are chlamydial culture negative and that CBC and sedimentation rates are normal (see Sections #11 and #16). These procedures are performed on approximately the eighth day of the menstrual cycle, with perioperative antibiotic cover. The specific diagnosis of the tuboperitoneal disorder is ascertained after reviewing the data obtained from:

- Hystersalpingogram
- Hysteroscopy
- Laparoscopy
- Salpingoscopy (in selected cases)

Common diagnoses include:

- Healthy fimbriae with periovarian and/or peritubal adhesions
- Fimbrial adhesions
- Tubal phimosis
- Minor hydrosalpinx with some residual fimbria
- Dilated large hydrosalpinx with absence of fimbriae
- Proximal tubal occlusion
- Endometriosis
- Salpingitis isthmica nodosa
- Diverticuli of the proximal oviduct

Management

Currently, many patients with patent oviducts but associated scattered endometriosis, peritubal and/or periovarian adhesions and/or adhesions of various organs are treated at laparoscopy, using such operative endoscopic techniques as:

- Salpingolysis
- Ovariolysis
- Transection of adhesions between and/or among the:
  - Bowel
  - Ovary
  - Tube
  - Pelvic peritoneal surfaces

Scattered endometriosis is vaporized with the KTP-532, Argon, YAG or CO_2 laser.

Total Tubal Occlusion – Distal

A small, well-vascularized hydrosalpinx is managed by microsurgical salpingoneostomy.

Large dilated hydrosalpinges (greater than 3 cm in diameter) with absence of endosalpingeal folds on hysterosalpingogram or salpingoscopy are opened at laparoscopy, and the patient is offered IVF because of the poor prognosis for microsurgery.

Proximal Tubal Occlusion – Isthmic

Isthmic proximal tubal occlusion is suspected when endometriosis or salpingitis isthmica nodosa is present. These patients are treated with danazol (Danocrine® 400 mg bid) or GnRH agonist therapy. Repeat hysterosalpingogram two to four months later may reveal patency with resolution of the appearance of tubal diverticuli.

True proximal cornual tubal occlusion is treated with microsurgical cornual dissection and subsequent isthmo or ampullary cornual anastomosis.

Proximal tubal occlusion may be resolved by transuterine tubal probing and catheterization. If the lesion is considered to be an isolated solitary block, fluoroscopic ultrasound monitoring or operative hysteroscopy may be attempted. Tubal catheterization is carried out during preliminary diagnostic laparoscopy and hysteroscopy. If the procedure is unsuccessful and the patient has healthy distal oviducts (fimbriae), microsurgical tubal anastomosis may be considered.

Principles of Microsurgery

General

All data accumulated at hystersalpingogram, hysteroscopy and laparoscopy are combined, and the couple is counseled regarding:

- Diagnosis
- The overall microsurgical procedure

- The anticipated live birth rate from microsurgery (Table 22.1)
- The chances of possible ectopic pregnancy
- Alternative options, such as IVF

If the couple decides in favor of surgery, the procedure is scheduled for the mid-proliferative phase of the menstrual cycle (approximately day eight). Patients are administered perioperative antibiotics (second-generation cephalosporins 1 to 2 g or doxycycline 200 mg). Corticosteroids (eg, dexamethasone 20 mg intraperitoneal, 20 mg IM immediately after surgery and 10 mg IM at six hourly intervals) and Phenergan® 25 mg are given at six hourly intervals for 36 hours after surgery in an attempt to minimize adhesions.

Operative Procedure

The operative protocol is to:

- Place the patient in the lithotomy position
- Prepare the vagina, and drain the bladder using a Foley's catheter
- Grasp the cervix with a single-toothed tenaculum
- Sound the uterus to assess ease of entry and length of cavity (for possible future IVF)
- Insert an intrauterine catheter preloaded with dilute indigo carmine (this facilitates chromotubation in cases with tubal occlusion)
- Place a Kerlix pack, soaked in an antiseptic solution, in the vagina to elevate the uterus
  - No pack is used if:
    - Uterine retroversion is fixed
    - The possibility of multiple adhesions in the cul-de-sac is present
- Lower the patient's legs and place her in a supine position
- Prepare the abdomen, and drape it with a steri-drape
- Using a Pfannenstiel's incision, "split" the skin with a scalpel; transect all layers, using the electrocoagulator in a blend or coagulating mode. It is essential that blood be prevented from spilling

into the peritoneal cavity; this avoids fibrin deposition and, thereby, reduces the likelihood of subsequent adhesion formation

- Wash the glove talc from the hands before entering the peritoneal cavity
- Open the peritoneum, and infuse the abdomen with approximately 100 mL of an irrigation solution made of:
  - Ringer's lactate containing 2,000 IU heparin/L
  - 100 mg hydrocortisone/L
  - 100 mg ampicillin/L (pending patient sensitivity to penicillin)
- Apply a Kirschner retractor, and pack the bowel with lint-free lap sponges which have been soaked in the heparinized solution. All blades should be covered with similarly soaked lap sponges, and all intra-abdominal packs should be ring-tagged to ensure their removal
- Review the pelvis carefully and assess:
  - Adhesion sites
  - The need to mobilize adnexa from adjacent organs
  - The procedures needed to correct fimbrial gonadal relationships
- Excise and divide any adhesions, using an operative loupe with two- to four-fold magnification, to facilitate elevation of the adnexa
- Irrigate, using a Gomel irrigator
- Pack the cul-de-sac with lint-free Kerlix sponges to keep the tubes and ovaries close to the anterior abdominal wall
- Remove the loupe
- Bring the operating microscope into the field

Instrumentation, Operative Techniques and Methods

Checking the Microscope

Before beginning a microsurgical procedure, the surgeon and assistant should always check the focus of their eye pieces. Microsurgical dissection is accomplished with fine, micro-pickups and is assisted by a microelectrode or a sapphire-tipped YAG laser and microbipolar electrode. The tissues are to be irrigated continuously. When the dissection is completed, tissues requiring approximation are sutured using a micro needleholder-stitchcutter, or simple microsurgical needleholder, with the assistant using microscissors to cut suture ends.

Suture materials are usually of the 8-0, non-reactive variety; these include sutures made of polyglycolic acid and polylactic, polypropylene, polydioxan and monofilament nylon. All needles are tapered except for those used in anastomosis, which are of the "taper cut" variety. Ophthalmic cutting needles are not used because of their tendency to transect micro-vessels in the serosa and mesosalpinx.

Adhesion Prophylaxis

Surgeons may prevent adhesions by using gentle, atraumatic and meticulously hemostatic operative techniques and by ensuring that:

- The surgery is timed during the less vascular, mid-proliferative phase of the menstrual cycle
- The operating field is irrigated continuously during the procedure so that tissues are never allowed to desiccate (dry)
- Bleeding and deposition of fibrin on peritoneal surfaces is prevented by pinpoint hemostasis and heparinized irrigation
- Fluid is left in the pelvis after the procedure. This fluid is comprised of either:
    - 200 mL of the irrigation solution AND
    - 20 mg dexamethasone OR
    - 50 to 100 mL high molecular weight dextran
- The patient is nursed in a high Fowler's position for 36 to 48 hours to keep fluid in the cul-de-sac and to accomplish hydroflotation of the pelvic organs

Specific Operative Principles

The initial dissection, to excise gross adhesions and mobilize the adnexa, is usually completed using a loupe. Fine tissues (eg, fimbriae, isthmus and cornu) requiring more detailed dissection are elevated on Kerlix-soaked sponges.

The operating microscope is brought into the field, and the specific procedure is performed under proper magnification (six to 10 times).

Fimbrioplasty

The fimbriae are dissected, using the microelectrode or sapphire-tipped YAG laser scalpel. The ostium is then everted by using:

- A defocused laser beam (CO_2) OR
- 8-0 polyglycolic acid sutures, inserted at selected sites to ensure eversion of the fimbrial end of the oviduct

Salpingoneostomy

The central dimple of the occluded oviduct is defined and remnants of fimbrial folds are dissected under the operating microscope and everted using the techniques described for fimbrioplasty (see above).

Tubal Anastomosis

Detailed dissection of the proximal and distal occlusion sites are completed under the operating microscope. After adequate preparation, the two ends are sutured using 8-0 polyglycolic acid or polylactic suture material with taper-cut needles.

The usual suture order is from the 6 o'clock to the, 12, 3, and 9 o'clock positions. Muscularis is sutured to muscularis and serosa to serosa.

Prior to closure of the abdomen, the pelvis is inspected thoroughly. In selected patients, ventrosuspension, as a simple triplication of the round ligaments, is completed.

Ovarian Repair

For ovarian repair, 3-0 and 4-0 polydioxanone and polyglyconate sutures are placed within the ovary. 6-0, 7-0 polydioxanone and polyglyconate sutures are used on the surface of the ovary, ensuring that minimal suture is exposed to the outer surface of this organ.

Retrograde Tubal Irrigation

Retrograde tubal irrigation through a smooth, soft, rounded, tubal catheter facilitates division of intratubal adhesions.

Correction of Fimbrial Gonadal Derangement

If the tubal ostium is displaced from the ovarian surface by more than 4 cm, the fimbria ovarica is reconstructed using 7-0 polypropylene sutures.

Abdominal Closure

A continuous, 0 polyglycolic acid or polylactic, nonlocking suture is used for abdominal closure because it approximates the peritoneum. This compressed, watertight closure prevents leakage of the intraperitoneal fluid into the wound.

The fascia is closed with 0 synthetic absorbable suture in a continuous suture line and three to four additional interrupted sutures. The subcutaneous fat is closed with a 3-0 absorbable continuous suture, and the skin is approximated with a 4-0 subcuticular suture. Steri-strips are then applied.

This elaborate closure has rarely been associated with wound complications despite perioperative use of corticosteroids.

Postoperative Care

Postoperatively:

- The patient is nursed in a high Fowler's position for 36 to 48 hours
- IV fluids and intake/output (particularly those with dextran 70) are meticulously monitored

- The patient is monitored to avoid fluid overload and to check for pulmonary and/or allergic reactions
- The patient is given perioperative antibiotic therapy
- Corticosteroids and Phenergan® administered postoperatively
- The patient is discharged on the third or fourth postoperative day
- The patient is seen 10 to 14 days after surgery and then at six weeks
- The patient may resume sexual activity and automobile driving at three weeks after surgery and full regular physical activities at six weeks after surgery

Counseling – Time of Possible Pregnancy

With distal tubal disease, patients usually conceive from 10 months to three years or more after surgery; proximal tubal disease patients may conceive earlier, from three or four months to 18 months or two years after surgery. Conceptions occur early after restoration of proximal patency with normal fimbriae but are rare before the first year following distal tubal surgery (eg, salpingoneostomy).

All patients are counseled to see their physicians early in their pregnancies to exclude the possibility of tubal pregnancy.

Follow-Up

All patients are checked for adequacy of:

- Postcoital tests
- Ovulation
- Exclusion of secretory/luteal phase defect during long-term postoperative management

Postoperative – Hysterosalpingogram (HSG)

The postoperative hysterosalpingogram (HSG) is carried out at six months in those who have had complicated procedures. All others undergo HSG at one year, unless otherwise indicated.

Second-Look Laparoscopy

Second-look laparoscopy is performed primarily in patients with complicated myomectomy and/or periovarian surgery at six weeks to three months after surgery. The procedure is rarely necessary for those who submitted to microsurgical tubal anastomosis during the first year after surgery, since most patients conceive before that time.

HSG is often completed at one year to 18 months after other microsurgical procedures.

Comment

Routine second-look laparoscopy at six to eight weeks remains controversial since, when patients are reassessed two to three years after the original surgical procedure, there are no data to support a greater incidence of live births following early second-look laparoscopy.

On the other hand, clearly complicated procedures should be followed by early second-look laparoscopy. This provides a definitive assessment in cases of extremely poor outcome and avoids long-term follow-up. Such patients are better served by referral for early IVF.

Microsurgery vs. IVF

If a surgical procedure is expected to yield less than 20 percent live births, patients are often counseled toward IVF. If success rates are expected to be higher (ie, greater than 30 to 35 percent), patients may initially choose microsurgery and consider IVF if the procedure does not result in pregnancy.

When distal tubal occlusion occurs in patients over age 35, the usual, lengthy interval before pregnancy occurs may indicate the need for IVF, which, if successful, results in early pregnancy and avoids the stress associated with the "biological clock" time factor.

Table 22.1 – **Live Birth Rates for Tubal Microsurgery and Incidence of Ectopic Pregnancy**

	Live Birth Rate %	Ectopic Pregnancy Rate%
Salpingolysis/ Ovariolysis	40 to 70 %	5 to 10 %
Fimbriolysis	35 to 45 %	5 to 10%
Salpingoneostomy		
A. (Well vascularized, small oviduct with residual mucosa)	25 to 35%	10 to 17%
B. Large hydrosalpinx with absent mucosa	10 to 15%	10 to 25%
Proximal Tubal Occlusion (Previous sterilization)	60 to 80%	< 5%
Proximal Tubal Occlusion Pathological Cornual Occlusion	40 to 56%	3 to 10%
Tubal Reconstruction Congenital Anomalies	30 to 56%	< 5%

NOTES

#23 Endometriosis

Definition

Endometriosis is the presence of endometrial tissue at sites outside the endometrial cavity, including:

- Peritoneal surfaces
- Uterosacral ligaments
- Rectovaginal shelf
- Ovaries
- Bowel
- Ureter
- Distal sites, including:
  - Chest
  - Subcutaneous tissues

Associations

Endometriosis is associated with such factors as:

- Relatively thin females
- Postponed childbearing to later age
- Dynamic, tense, anxious career- or goal-oriented women
- Obsessive and perfectionistic dispositions
- Stressful lifestyles

It may also be associated with congenital anomalies of the genital tract which obstruct menses, including cervical stenosis and all causes of obstructions of the:

- Uterus
- Cervix
- Vagina

Endometriosis is sometimes linked to DES exposure.

Theories of Origin

Endometriosis may be due to:

- Retrograde menstruation
- Coelomic metaplasia
- Lymphatic spread
- Hematogenous spread

It can spread directly by continuity and contiguity (classically seen after previous uterine operative procedures).

Clinical Presentation

Patients with endometriosis will likely present with:

- Dysmenorrhea, pelvic pain
- Dyspareunia
- Bladder and/or bowel disturbances at menses associated with nausea and sensations of hotness and coldness
- Intermittent lower abdominal pain
- Infertility
- Menstrual irregularities, including:
  - Premenstrual spotting
  - Postmenstrual spotting
  - Mid-cycle spotting
- Hypomenorrhea or menorrhagia

Patients may be asymptomatic, being diagnosed at laparoscopy or laparotomy performed for a different reason, or they may present with such complications as rupture or hemorrhage of the endometrioma.

Endometrial tissue growth may range from minor spots on peritoneal surfaces to masses involving large endometriomas (greater than 10 cm). Endometrial tissue may include solid involvement and fixity of the bladder and bowel or massive infiltration of uterosacral ligaments, mimicking cervical carcinoma.

Diagnosis

Diagnosis of endometriosis is made by:

- History
- Physical examination
- Hysterosalpingogram
- Laparoscopy

Factors to be noted in the history include:

- Overall disposition and patient profile (see Section #7)
- Occurrence of:
  - Infertility
  - Pelvic pain
  - Dysmenorrhea
  - Dyspareunia

- Menstrual abnormalities with a relative temperature rise during menses (this is likely to be related to retrograde menstruation and absorption of blood products from the pelvic cavity)

Factors to be noted in the physical examination include:

- Weight—Low body weight or associated low body fat. Commonly, such women have fibroadenosis of the breasts
- Spots of endometriosis on the cervix
- Abnormal cervix and possible obstructive element
- Pelvis with endometriosis, ranging from normal to tender palpable uterosacral ligaments and/or pelvic masses (endometriomas)
- Access to the uterosacral ligaments via pelvirectal exam; with this, endometriosis can frequently be diagnosed at its earliest stage

If endometriosis is present, the hysterosalpingogram will usually demonstrate:

- Open tubes
- Convoluted oviducts or saccular dilatation with distortion and displacement of oviducts
- Proximal oviduct pathology resembling salpingitis isthmica nodosa

Laparoscopy offers documentation, diagrams, photography, video recording and classification according to the American Fertility Society (See Section #16), as well as biopsy for histological confirmation.

Reasons for Infertility

The reasons for infertility due to endometriosis are unknown but may be linked to:

- Dysfunction of hypothalamic-pituitary-gonadal axis
- Pelvic pain due to dyspareunia and/or infrequency of intercourse
- Ovulatory disorders, including:
    - Inadequate ovulation
    - Inadequate LH surges with luteinized unruptured follicle syndrome, AND/OR

- Luteal phase defect and discrepancies with low plasma progesterone
    - Out-of-phase endometrial biopsy
- Poor cervical mucus and inadequate postcoital tests with poor sperm penetration due to a relative hypoestrogenic status
- Release of prostaglandins from lesions and retrograde menstrual fluid, causing derangements of functions of oviducts and tubal secretions
- Macrophages and histiocytes related to possible phagocytosis of sperm or creation of an abnormal environment precluding fertilization
- Possible derangement of oviducts' and ovarys' special relationships, resulting from elongation of the fimbria ovarica with displacement of the tubal ostium well away from the ovarian surface
- True mechanical derangements, with adhesions causing:
    - Tubal occlusion or relative phimosis
    - Tuboperitoneal adhesions
    - Tubo-ovarian adhesions
    - Periovarian adhesions/endometriosis
- Ovarian involvement with endometriomas and associated endocrine and ovulatory disturbances
- Immunological mechanisms

Principles of Management

Endometriosis may be managed by:

- Operative endoscopy, ie, laser vaporization, at diagnostic operative laparoscopy
- CO_2 laser
- KTP-532 laser
- Argon laser
- Sapphire-tipped YAG laser
- Medical therapy

The regimen of medical therapy after laparoscopic diagnosis is:

- Danazol therapy (Danocrine® 400 mg twice daily) for three to eight months, depending on the extent and severity of endometriosis, OR

- Danazol therapy (Danocrine® 400 mg twice daily) for three months prior to conservative surgery for pelvic endometriosis, OR
- GnRH agonist therapy (Lupron® 0.5 to 1 mg daily or Synarel® [nafarelin acetate] 400 μg daily intranasally) for three to four months, depending on the extent of the disease
- Medroxyprogesterone acetate (Provera® 5 to 20 mg daily) for three to six months

Conservative Surgery

Pelvic endometriosis may be managed by conservative surgery, including:

- Bilateral salpingolysis
- Bilateral ovariolysis
- Laser vaporization
- Laser vaporization and dissection of endometriomas with ovarian reconstruction and uterosacral ablation
- Presacral neurectomy

Expectant Management

Treatment of associated ovulatory dysfunctions, such as supplemented ovulation induction, is by:

- Clomiphene citrate plus HCG
- Clomiphene citrate plus HCG plus bromocriptine plus or minus dexamethasone
- HMG plus HCG
- Progesterone vaginal suppositories for those with diagnosed secretory/luteal phase defect
- IVF or GIFT procedure

Additional Therapeutic Choices

For patients in whom above therapies have failed to result in conception, other therapeutic options exist.

Mild endometriosis may be managed by:

- Laser vaporization, chromotubation and pelvic irrigation
- Supplemented ovulation induction following laser laparoscopy

- Danazol therapy (Danocrine® 800 mg daily [400 mg twice a day]) for three months, OR
- GnRH agonist therapy (Lupron® or Synarel®) for three months, followed by expectant management or supplemented ovulation induction
- Medroxyprogesterone acetate therapy (Provera® 5 to 20 mg daily) for three to six months

Moderate endometriosis may be managed by:

- Laser laparoscopy drainage and removal of pelvic endometriomas by mass pelvic irrigation
- Laser ablation of uterosacral ligaments in those with dysmenorrhea, followed by:
  - Danazol (Danocrine® 400 mg twice daily) for four months post-surgery OR
  - GnRH agonist (Lupron® 0.5 to 1 mg daily or Synarel® [nafarelin acetate] 400 μg intranasally daily) for four months post-surgery

These patients should consider a second laparoscopy, with expectant management and/or supplemented ovulation induction.

Severe endometriosis and/or failure of above therapies to successfully treat moderate endometriosis may be managed by:

- Preoperative suppression of endometriosis with danazol (Danocrine® 400 mg twice daily) for three to four months, OR
- Preoperative suppression with GnRH agonists (Lupron® 0.5 to 1 mg daily or Synarel® [nafarelin acetate] 400 μg intranasally daily) for three to four months
- Post-suppression conservative surgery, including:
  - Laparotomy
  - Resection of multiple intrapelvic adhesions
  - Bilateral salpingolysis
  - Bilateral ovariolysis
  - Resection of the residual endometriomas with ovarian reconstruction
  - Presacral neurectomy and/or, if marked dysmenorrhea, uterosacral ablation

- Ventrosuspension
- Retrograde chromotubation
- Microsurgical correction of distal tubal anomalies:
  - If one ovary has been damaged by extensive pathology, it should be resected and the healthy tube and ovary conserved
  - If the tube on the oophorectomy side is healthy, it should be transposed to the remaining healthy contralateral ovary (if feasible)
  - Postoperative continuation of danazol (Danocrine®) and/or GnRH agonist (Lupron® or Synarel®), depending on the severity and extent of the pathology and the ability to surgically remove all endometriosis

NOTE: Lupron® may be given in a long-acting monthly dose of 7.5 mg IM.

Whenever possible, medical suppression of endometriosis with danazol or GnRH agonists is preferable to major resection of the bowel, bladder and/or ureter. These radical surgical procedures are ideally deferred until after childbearing, unless indicated for emergency reasons, such as impending bowel or ureteric obstruction. In rare but selected cases, patients may undergo marked suppression and major surgery for endometriosis followed by early consideration for postoperative IVF because of extensive oviduct destruction (noted at surgery).

In all cases, if above therapies fail after a reasonable treatment period (ie, 12 to 18 months), patients should consider an IVF or GIFT procedure.

Anticipated Prognosis

The prognosis for pregnancy and live birth after 18 months to three years for all modalities of therapy are approximately:

- 70 percent for mild endometriosis
- 45 to 50 percent for moderate endometriosis
- 35 to 40 percent for severe endometriosis

The prognosis is also age-dependent, with fewer older patients conceiving; therefore, diagnosis should be established early and treatment should begin in a timely fashion.

Possible Prevention

Fifty percent of teenagers presenting with recurrent abdominal pain and/or dysmenorrhea have endometriosis. Diagnostic laparoscopy should be considered early in the management of these patients. After diagnosis, danazol should be instituted for adequate suppression of estradiol levels and birth control pills (OCs) should be given for suppression maintenance. During danazol therapy, if estradiol is not adequately suppressed to less than 30 pg/mL, subsequent GnRH agonist therapy is indicated for four to six months. This is followed by OC maintenance therapy.

Patients in this age group should be counseled to consider childbirth soon after marriage if they seriously desire children.

Precautions Regarding Danazol Therapy

Though side effects of danazol (Danocrine®) therapy have been observed, patients who have been adequately counseled prior to therapy do not commonly experience them.

Because danazol is begun during menstruation, there is minimal risk of pregnancy. The initial dosage is 200 mg twice daily for 10 days (during which time the patient is to use mechanical contraception), followed by the standard dose of 400 mg twice a day for three to six months, depending on the stage of the disease.

Once the patient's therapy is established, a SMAC profile should be performed at six weekly intervals to diagnose changes in hepatic enzymes and blood lipids. To alleviate muscle cramps, patients should be given supplemental calcium during therapy.

In view of the androgenic properties and possible adverse effects of danazol on plasma lipids, patients should be counseled to avoid high-cholesterol foods.

After four to six weeks of therapy, a plasma estradiol should be drawn; if estradiol is above 30 ng/mL (indicating failure of adequate suppression of the hypothalamic-pituitary axis), GnRH agonist therapy should be considered.

If breakthrough bleeding occurs during danazol therapy, patients should be given a short course of conjugated estrogens. The regimen is:

- 0.625 mg tid for three days, FOLLOWED BY
- 0.625 mg bid for three days, FOLLOWED BY
- 0.625 mg once daily for three days

This will usually alleviate bleeding for at least six weeks and facilitate continuance of danazol therapy.

Patients must be counseled regarding increased appetite during therapy. With conscientious weight-watching, however, patients will not necessarily gain weight.

When danazol therapy is discontinued, patients should use mechanical contraception for two weeks before attempting conception. This interval allows time for adequate endometrium to develop so that, upon ovulation, conception may be facilitated and implantation and placental formation may be normal.

GnRH Agonist Therapy

GnRH agonist therapy (Lupron® Injection/Synarel® Intranasal Spray) may be administered in an injectable preparation daily or monthly or in alternate delivery systems, such as a nasal spray form. The mechanism of action of the GnRH agonist is down regulation of pituitary gondadotropins, resulting in low levels of FSH and LH and, consequently, hypogonadotropic hypogonadism.

Early reports of GnRH agonist therapy for producing a reversible, true menopausal state indicate results equivalent to and, in some circumstances, better than danazol but with a loss of anabolic effects and a major shifting of bone calcium. Recent data indicate that prophylactic administration of calcium of 1 to 1.5 g daily during administration of GnRH agonist may prevent bone loss. A positive effect is the maintenance of normal lipid values, with no adverse changes in HDL and LDL cholesterol levels.

Classic side effects of GnRH agonists are:

- Hot flashes
- Headaches
- Irritability
- Insomnia

Many patients prefer these side effects to the potential androgenic side effects of danazol.

The major theoretical side effect of GnRH preparations is the possible induction of GnRH antibodies, which may result in a loss of normal cyclic activity of the patient's own GnRH and cause:

- Menstrual irregularity
- Ovulatory dysfunction
- Infertility

In view of the small size of the GnRH molecule, this risk of antibody stimulation is considered to be very low.

The major indication for GnRH agonists in young patients is a failure of danazol therapy to result in adequate lowering of estradiol. If this occurs, GnRH can be added to the regimen and danazol withdrawn; the hypogonadotropic hypogonadal state facilitates atrophy of the endometriosis. In patients over age 30, danazol and GnRH agonists should be given equal consideration, with administration dependent on individual case assessment.

Endometriosis and Surgical Lasers

The objective of using surgical lasers to treat endometriosis is to vaporize the endometriosis without destroying adjacent tissues.

The CO_2 Laser

The CO_2 laser is a non-visible, high-wavelength laser which is guided by columnization with helium neon (the "red spot" beam). Fifteen to 40 watts are used at abdominal laparotomy and three to 10 watts at laparoscopy. The pulse beam is at 0.05 to 1 per second; a super pulse mode is used for cutting.

The CO_2 laser has a major role in intra-abdominal vaporization of periovarian and peritoneal endometriosis. It has minimal depth of penetration; therefore, actual vaporization is visualized as it occurs, and no damage beyond the visible tissue being vaporized occurs.

The CO_2 laser is used extensively via the operating laparoscopic single puncture (mobilizing organs through the second puncture) or second puncture (in a double-puncture technique).

Particular caution must be taken during use of the continuous mode. Back-stops and nonreflective surfaces are required, since the CO_2 laser can accidentally be reflected from shiny surfaces and burn distant organs.

Intensive training is necessary for the totally effective and safe laparoscopic use of the CO_2 laser.

The KTP-532 Fiberoptic Laser

The KTP-532 (potassium titanyl phosphate crystal) fiberoptic laser passes a YAG laser beam through a KTP-532 crystal, halving the wave length from 1064 to 532. Because the greenish-blue beam appears within the spectrum of human vision, no aiming beam is used with the KTP-532 laser. The laser defocuses within a centimeter of the fiberoptic; depth of penetration is 1 to 2 mm beyond the focal point.

The KTP-532 laser has a relatively selective photo absorption and, therefore, is a very effective means of treating dark red or black deposits of endometriosis.

The major use of the KTP-532 is in laparoscopy; it has virtually no use or advantage in intra-abdominal surgery at open laparotomy. It may be used through the operating channel or a second-puncture channel and is particularly safe in laparoscopy because of its limited depth of penetration. Because the laser is completely defocused within millimeters of the fiber, there is minimal risk of reflection injuries.

The learning curve for students of the KTP-532 fiberoptic laser is relatively fast, and the technique is easily reproducible, requiring less training than that necessary for CO_2 laser use through the laparoscope.

The KTP-532 may be used for transection of adhesions, vaporization of pelvic endometriosis and drainage of endometriomas.

The Argon Fiberoptic Laser

The Argon laser is used as a fiberoptic system. It has a bluish color within the wave length of human vision and a relative depth of penetration of 1 to 2 mm. Its definite photo absorption makes it highly effective for laparoscopic vaporization of peritoneal, periovarian and intrapelvic endometriosis.

YAG Laser

The main use of the YAG laser is as a fiberoptic for intrauterine endometrial ablation and/or division of a uterine septum. Its depth of penetration beyond visualized vaporization is up to 4 mm. The YAG laser is not used as a bare fiber in laparoscopy, though, theoretically, it can be used at very low wattage (eg, 2 to 3 watts).

Major laparoscopic use of the YAG laser is with a sapphire tip for gynecological microsurgery and dissection of adhesions from tube and tubal tissues. The sapphire-tipped fiberoptic YAG laser has excellent applications via the laparoscope. Varying the sapphire tip shapes affords different actions; the "touch technique" facilities the YAG laser's relatively simple and safe application via the laparoscope.

#24 Immunological Infertility: Antisperm Antibodies

Immunological infertility implies failure of conception due to the presence of sperm-agglutinating and sperm-immobilizing antibodies. These may be of the immunoglobin class of either IgG, IgA or IgM.

Sperm antibodies have presented multiple problems with respect to their diagnosis and treatment. Indeed, the possibility of antibodies to the sperm's surface, acrosome or inner contents have presented diagnostic difficulties in their interpretation with respect to their clinical significance and therapeutic import.

There are many methods of assessing sperm antibodies, including sperm-agglutinating and sperm-immobilizing tests. Recently, however, the use of antibody-coated microspheres to assess antisperm antibodies of IgG, IgA and IgM globulins to the sperm head, neck or tail have facilitated a highly-specific sperm antibody test. Furthermore, the sperm immunobead antibody test provides a quantitative assessment of the percentage of sperm possessing such antibodies.

Sperm antibodies may be measured in:

- Serum
- Cervical mucus
- Seminal fluid
- Washed spermatozoa

Antibodies of the IgG class are far more significant than those of the IgA class, which in turn are more significant than those of the IgM class. Additionally, antibodies to the sperm head are more sinister than those against the sperm tail.

In the female, the antibodies may express themselves in the serum and cervical mucus; and, although difficult to assess, they may act negatively as transudates of the uterine or oviduct fluids.

In the male, sperm antibodies may be measured in the serum, seminal plasma or the sperm itself. Significant antibodies may attack the outer membranes of the sperm head, neck or tail.

Causes of Sperm Antibodies

In the female, antibodies are an uncommon response to the deposition of semen within the vagina. Sensitization may occur, however, and there is some evidence that this may be linked to breach of the genital mucosa by infection or menstruation.

The antibodies may be of a general or local variety. It is important to recall that the patient may have high levels of serum antibodies yet low levels locally in the cervical mucus. By contrast, there may be low levels of systemic serum antibodies associated with high levels of cervical mucus antisperm antibodies.

In the male, antisperm antibodies are usually associated with oligo- or normospermia; but when seen with severe oligospermia or azoospermia, this suggests the possibility of gonadal destruction in an autoimmune dysfunction.

This may be associated with viral orchitis and a breach in the blood/testis or blood/semen barrier. A breach in the blood/semen barrier may occur in the testicle or the collecting duct system of the rete testis, epididymis or vas deferens.

The classic example of this occurs following a vasectomy in which a pressure breach of the epididymis or vas may result in semen and spermatozoa leaking into the systemic circulation. This process results in sensitization and formation of antisperm antibodies.

Antisperm antibodies may be seen in cases having had previous vasectomy, inguinoscrotal surgery, infection or inflammation, including:

- Prostatitis
- Epididymitis
- Orchitis
- Testicular injuries
- Idiopathic causes

Antisperm antibodies should also be suspected in cases of hyperspermia (counts greater than 150 million per mL).

Clinical Presentation

Antisperm antibodies may affect five percent of couples presenting with infertility. Presentation may include:

- Poor cervical mucus
- Impenetrable yet normal-appearing cervical mucus
- Recurrent abnormal postcoital tests associated with agglutination and/or immobilization of sperm
- Shaking movements of the sperm within the cervical mucus
- Head-to-head or tail-to-tail agglutination
- Recurrent absence of sperm in the cervical mucus
- Immobilized sperm within the cervical mucus

Another presentation is that of idiopathic infertility which is accompanied by apparently normal postcoital tests and having found no abnormality to explain the infertility.

Pathophysiology

Antibodies affect fertility by:

- Preventing sperm's penetration of cervical mucus
- Immobilizing sperm in the female genital tract
- Preventing sperm penetration of the ovum
- Destroying sperm within the oviduct

In the male, antisperm antibodies may coat the sperm and prevent its normal function at any stage of its passage through the female genital tract.

Clinical Tests

A diagnosis of antisperm antibodies is suggested by:

- Recurrent abnormal postcoital tests
- Shaky movements of sperm within the cervical mucus
- Head-to-head or tail-to-tail sperm agglutination
- Multiple immobilized sperm, though the male has apparent "normal" semen analysis and the female has "perfect" cervical mucus

Crossmatch testing employs the use of donor sperm and donor mucus to assess if the apparent antisperm antibody is due to a "hostile" mucus or a sperm component (Figure 12.2).

Diagnosis

If antibodies appear to be present in screening tests (eg, crossmatch testing with donor sperm and donor mucus), it is advisable to complete an immunobead sperm antibody test.

IgG, IgA, IgM Immunobead Antibody Test

The immunobead antibody test is performed during the female's proliferative phase of the menstrual cycle. Her cervical mucus is aspirated, blood is obtained from both partners and a fresh masturbatory sample of sperm is immediately fractionated into spermatozoa. (Fractionated semen is assessed separately for the presence or absence of sperm antibodies and for the direction of sperm antibodies [ie, against the sperm head, neck or tail], if present).

The results are recorded, together with the screening of the semen analysis, indicating the percentile of sperm antibodies present in serum, cervical mucus, semen or sperm and their classification. The antibody report is to be discussed with the patient (Table 24.1).

General Prognosis

The prognosis for fertility of a couple with antisperm antibodies is dependent on the severity (percentage) of antibodies present and the correlation of clinical with laboratory data. In certain circumstances, clinical sperm penetrability may appear better than that from the laboratory report (eg, 35 to 40 percent antibodies present of IgA, IgG, IgM class yet active sperm penetration in the postcoital test). Approximately 35 percent of these couples achieve conception with treatment.

If the presence of antibodies is above the 80th percentile of IgA, IgG, IgM (not uncommon in those with vasectomies of more than 10 years), pregnancies are rarely achieved without assisted reproductive technology (ART), ie, GIFT or IVF.

Therapeutic Concepts

Male

For the male with sperm antibodies, ideally spermatogenesis is suppressed by mass doses of testosterone along with a long or short course of corticosteroids.

For prolonged suppression, rebound therapy is probably not acceptable in current practice.

The alternatives are the use of corticosteroids. Prednisolone, for example, may be given 15 to 20 mg daily for three to six months (long-term therapy) or 96 mg daily, with reducing doses during the first 12 days of the female partner's menstrual cycle (short-term therapy). The high-dose, short-term, cyclic method has met with some success during the last decade.

The use of high doses of corticosteroids implies careful case selection and close monitoring to avoid gastric ulceration, bone destruction and the severe metabolic consequences of high-dose corticosteroid therapy. In recent years, short-term use of large doses of corticosteroids appears to have become favored, but extreme caution must be taken when using this technique.

In addition to medical therapy, the couple may undergo the local treatment method of washed sperm intrauterine insemination (WIUI) (see Section #28), completed at the time of ovulation. For this, sperm is washed and prepared in the routine manner, but washing is commenced immediately after ejaculation so that separation of sperm and seminal plasma antibodies may be completed as soon as possible. Washed insemination is then combined with controlled ovarian stimulation of the female partner. Data suggest that the highest success rate of fertility is accomplished by combining human menopausal gonadotropin (HMG) stimulation of the female with WIUI. The success rate is approximately 14 to 20 percent per cycle, with 25 to 40 percent of couples attaining conception over three to four treatment cycles.

In the event that the above relatively simple methods fail or if extremely high percentiles of antisperm antibodies in the male are present (ie, greater than 80 percent IgG, IgA or IgM), ART in the forms of IVF or GIFT, may be used. ART has met with definite success in recent years.

Female

Antisperm antibodies present in the female are treated similarly to those in the male. Treatment includes:

- Prolonged nonexposure to spermatozoa via condom therapy for a minimum of six to nine months
- Short-term corticosteroid therapy, administered during the first half of the menstrual cycle (this appears to be the least invasive, safest and most acceptable method of treatment)
- Controlled ovarian hyperstimulation in the female using:
  - Clomiphene citrate plus HCG OR
  - HMG plus HCG, together with *carefully-timed* WIUI of preincubated, prepared sperm (preferable)

General Assessment

Antisperm antibodies are responsible for infertility in approximately three to seven percent of couples. This significant factor must be sought in all couples presenting with idiopathic infertility and/or recurrent abnormal postcoital tests.

The overall prognosis for antisperm antibodies with all methods of therapy has been 35 percent successful gestations. However, research is presently being completed to improve this prognosis.

The mere findings of antisperm antibodies, even with failure of conception, is often very gratifying for the couple seeking a cause for their inability to reproduce. Discovering antisperm antibodies can be a welcome relief for those who have been frustrated by persistent counseling that "there is nothing wrong with them." Significant progress using ART has been made, but it is hoped that further advances in the field will facilitate conception in those who presently suffer from this immunological reproductive disorder about which relatively little is known.

Table 24.1 – **Sperm Antibody Test Results**

Patient Name ____________________

Referring Physician ____________ Date __________

*Immunobead Sperm Antibody Test**

HUSBAND:

	Washed Sperm % Positive	Seminal Fluid % Positive	Serum % Positive
IgA	______	______	______
IgG	______	______	______
IgM	______	______	______

WIFE:

	Cervical Mucus % Positive	Serum % Positive
IgA	______	______
IgG	______	______
IgM	______	______

Comments

Semen Analysis: ____________________

____

Sperm Antibody Test: ____________________

____

Abbreviations: H = Head
M = Midpiece
TPP = Tail Principle Piece
TT = Tail Tip

*If results are greater than 20%, refer to individual worksheets for complete breakdown.

#25 Idiopathic Infertility

Introduction

Idiopathic infertility implies the inability to diagnose a causative factor for failure of conception in a particular couple. The incidence of this diagnosis (usually about five percent of all couples investigated) is inversely proportional to the depth and meticulous detail applied to investigation of the couple.

Clinical Presentation

A diagnosis of indiopathic infertility is made after all other factors have been meticulously reviewed, evaluated and excluded as a possible cause of infertility.

An idiopathic infertile male will present with:

- No stress
- Normal semen analysis parameters and postcoital tests, confirmed by repeated examinations
- Normal hamster egg penetration assay
- No sperm antibodies

An idiopathic infertile female will present with:

- No stress
- Normal endocrine status with normal postcoital tests
- Adequate ovulation, confirmed by blood progesterones and repeated endometrial biopsy
- Normal uterine cavity, oviducts and pelvis, assessed radiologically and at:
  - Endoscopy
  - Hysteroscopy
  - Laparoscopy
  - Chromopertubation
- Normal ovaries, healthy ovarian surfaces and normal close relationships between fimbrial ostia and the ovaries
- Absence of antisperm antibodies

Patient Counseling

The clinician should confirm the current idiopathic failure of conception and offer the couple a review of assisted reproductive technology (ART) options, from the least to the most invasive of methods.

Management

If the couple wishes to pursue therapy, the first option is to supplement ovulation induction with clomiphene citrate and HCG and to perform washed sperm intrauterine insemination (WIUI). In this case, adequacy of cervical mucus and luteal phase endometrial biopsy is essential to avoid converting the cause of infertility from idiopathic to iatrogenic clomiphene citrate abuse. If cervical mucus and luteal phase are positive, the technique should be repeated three times. Approximately 15 percent of these patients conceive with this therapy.

If results are negative, the next therapeutic option involves HMG therapy, with adequate monitoring by ultrasound and E_2 (see Section #20) for ovulation induction.

WIUI and supplementation of the luteal phase with intramuscular or vaginal progesterone may be repeated three times. Twenty to 30 percent of these patients conceive with this therapy.

Failure of these methods indicates ART options.

IVF/GIFT/Combination Therapy/ZIFT

There are advantages and disadvantages of all ART methods.

IVF

Advantages of IVF (*in vitro* fertilization) (Figure 25.1) are that:

- Vaginal egg retrieval is less invasive than that of GIFT
- Fertilization can be observed
- Sperm-egg penetration can be confirmed

Disadvantages of IVF are that:

- There are continued difficulties in reproducing adequate laboratory IVF backup
- IVF is a difficult technique to reproduce

- IVF must be done in a facility with a proven record of viable pregnancies
- IVF's overall success rate is only about 15 to 20 percent per cycle

GIFT

The advantages of GIFT (gamete intrafallopian transfer) (Figure 25.2) are that:

- It is easy to reproduce with adequately-trained laboratory staff in adequately-equipped laboratories adjacent to operating rooms
- It has a higher success rate than IVF, since the clinician can rely on normal:
  - Physiology of the tubal environment
  - Cyclic timing
  - Mechanism of tubal transfer of morula to endometrial cavity

Disadvantages of GIFT are that:

- It is a blind procedure regarding confirmation of fertilization
- It requires laparoscopy or laparotomy for visualization and catheterization of the distal ends of the oviducts
- Pregnancy occurs in 25 to 40 percent of couples

Combination Therapy

Some couples choose to combine the GIFT and IVF procedures. This combination therapy enables confirmation of egg fertilization and allows couples to take advantage of:

- Additional oocytes harvested at IVF and transferred into the uterus during the same cycle OR
- Cryopreservation of embryos for transfer to the uterus at a later cycle

ZIFT

The ZIFT (zygote into fallopian tube) method (Figure 25.3) is a double-operative procedure currently under review. If it is proven to be superior to the above methods, it may have specific applications for couples with significant male factors.

The ZIFT procedure (see Section #30) requires:

- Initial transvaginal retrieval of oocytes
- Fertilization by prepared sperm in a Petri dish
- Confirmation of fertilization and observation of the zygote
- Laparoscopy and transfer of the ZIFT

The overall results of IVF are proportional to the number of times a patient undergoes a treatment cycle. In principle, the couple is counseled regarding repeated treatment (two to three times) to afford a reasonable (about 30 to 40 percent) chance of success.

Comment on Treatment Independent Pregnancy

Idiopathic infertile couples may experience normal conception regardless of treatment method failures and/or between "treatment" cycles (treatment independent pregnancy [TIP]). Couples should be adequately counseled to be aware of this possibility. The impact of the psychological factors, which are presently poorly understood, must never be underestimated.

If all methods fail and/or if patients choose to discontinue treatment, adoption is a further option that couples should be made aware of. If couples desire adoption, clinicians/counselors should refer them to the proper sources and offer further assistance as needed.

Figures 25.1, 25.2 and 25.3 ➡

FIGURE 25.1 – **IVF Procedure**

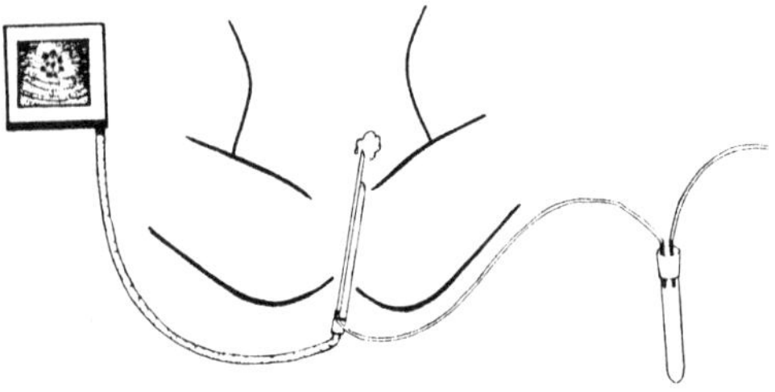

1. Vaginal egg retrieval using sonographic directed needle

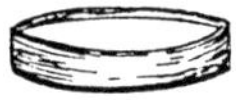

2. Incubation and fertilization *in vitro.* Eggs fertilized and cleavage within approximately 48 hours

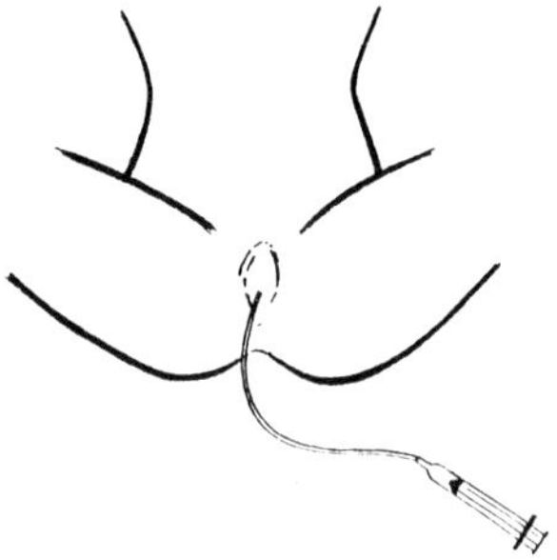

3. Transcervical embryo transfer to . . .

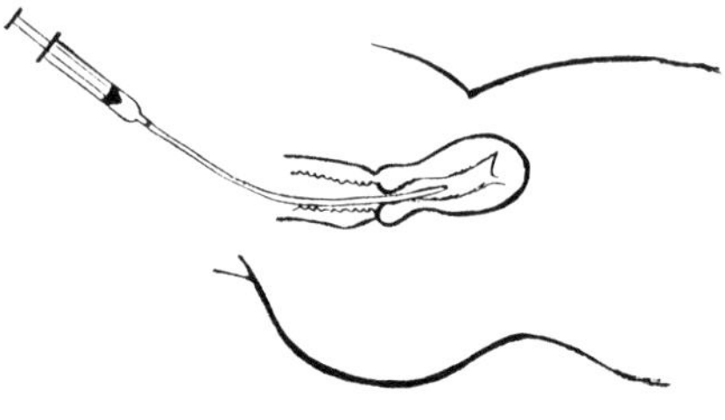

. . . uterus.

FIGURE 25.2 – **GIFT Procedure**

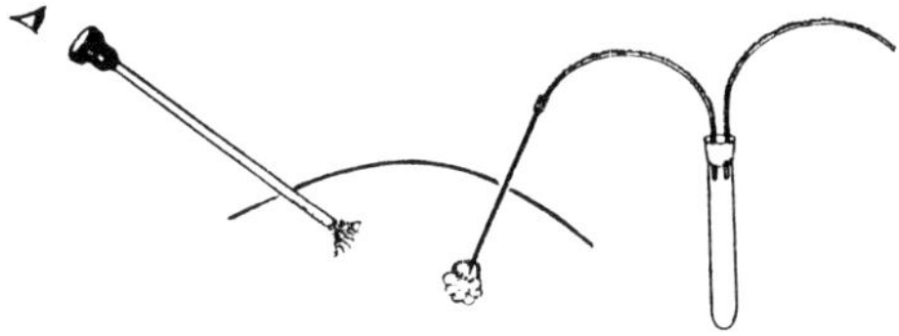

1. Laparoscopic egg retrieval

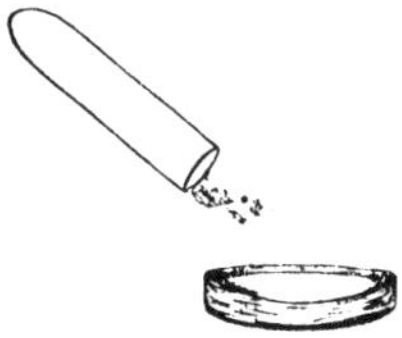

2. Harvested ova to culture medium

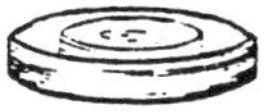

3. Preparation of semen

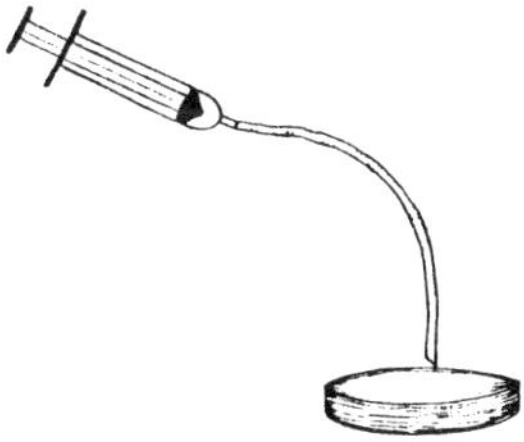

4. Catheter loaded sperm plus ova (approximately 3 per tube)

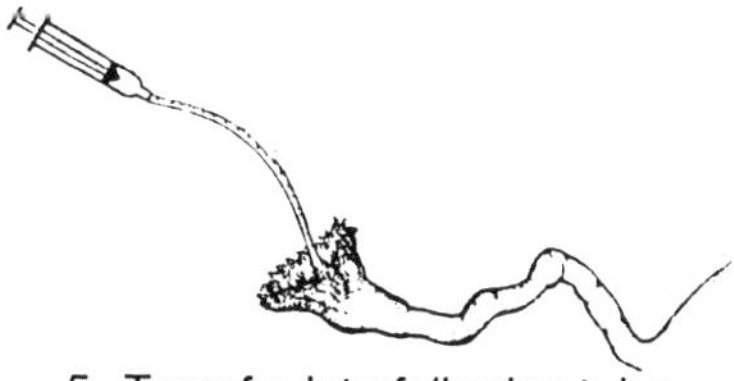

5. Transfer into fallopian tube

FIGURE 25.3 – **ZIFT/TET Procedure**

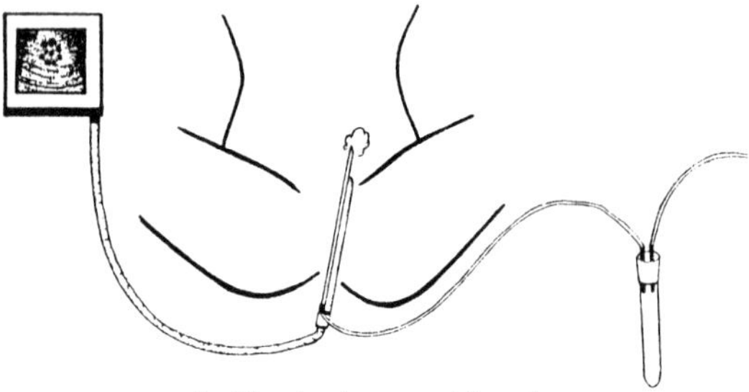

1. Vaginal egg retrieval

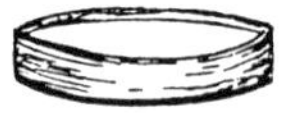

2. Incubation and fertilization *in vitro*

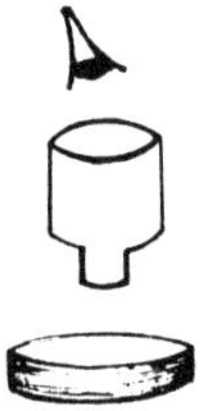

3. Confirm fertilization 24 to 36 hours

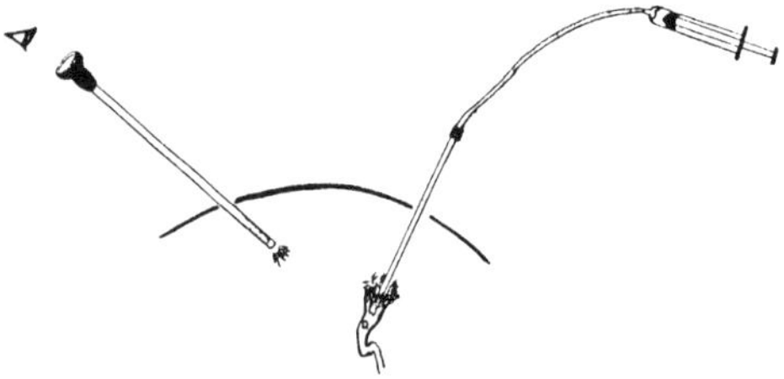

4. Laparoscopy and intratubal transfer of embryo (TET) or zygote (ZIFT)

NOTES

#26 Cessation of Treatment: The Adoption Option

Introduction

The impact and burden of the investigation and treatment of infertility is intense for all couples, and the situation is not only a physical and emotional burden but also a costly one in terms of time, energy and strain on the marriage and financial status. Both partners of a couple must cope with and work through the possibility that they may never conceive their own biological child, and this fact can have various impacts on individuals.

Some patients, especially those who never intended to be parents, show only relatively mild sadness and mourning at failure to conceive. Others, for whom childlessness impacts greatly, may experience major devastation unequalled by any other disaster they face, including the loss of a close relative.

Just as the decision to commence investigation and treatment for infertility is a major one, the decision to cease active attempts at conception can be an emotional trauma. This reaction can be minimized and possibly prevented if the clinician/counselor will honestly and adequately counsel couples regarding the course of investigation and treatments to be pursued; the relatively long months or years that treatment may require; and the fact that, after undergoing involved therapy, the goal of childbearing may still be denied.

From the first visit, couples should be made aware of various prognoses of fertility, specific therapeutic options and all facts regarding their case. The possibility that couples may never conceive or secure a healthy gestation must be reviewed at timely intervals, and the subject or consideration of adoption should never come as a sudden surprise or shock.

Negative reactions to treatment failures and/or cessation of treatment can be minimized or avoided if counseling is provided at all stages by:

- Physicians
- Office staff
- Counselors (usually clinical psychologists)

Adequate communication with families and friends is a must, and all support groups should be sensitive to the problem and avoid pressuring couples regarding their childless status.

The impact and positive effects of emotional support from these and other counselors (clergymen and support groups, such as RESOLVE) cannot be underestimated. Well-informed counselors who are adequately aware of the problem, its scientific basis and the need for emotional and spiritual support are an important part of a couple's need for and ability to participate in treatment. During couples' early visits, information about reproductive anatomy and physiology, principles of diagnoses, options of therapy and the potential duration of treatment must be communicated. Myths must also be expelled.

Throughout treatment, patients must be counseled and supported if and when they experience feelings of shock, guilt, denial, anger, punishment and/or total loss of control of their situation. The expected prognosis must be adequately communicated to patients, and the possibility of cessation of further treatment must be reviewed and reinforced intermittently.

No couple has a 100-percent guarantee of becoming pregnant and/or of delivering a healthy, live infant. This fact must be presented to, dealt with and resolved by each patient. Each couple must ask and answer the question, "What if we never have our much wanted child?" In answering this question, partners must be counseled not to place fault or apportion blame and instead to be mutually aware of each other's sensitivities and needs for emotional support.

Regrettably, a significantly large percentage of couples will not cope well with the stresses imposed by the problem of infertility. Some couples will divorce despite counseling and their efforts to cope. Occasionally, couples will separate during early stages of treatment once it is evident that one partner is sterile; such a decision may reflect a value system or cultural situation in which biological reproduction is demanded of a partner and a fertile partner may be forced to search for an alternate, fertile mate. (In its most primitive form, this thinking occurs in situations in which a man must impregnate his intended bride before a marriage is sanctioned. If the female does not conceive, an alternate female partner is chosen and married if she is fortunate to conceive. This thinking is not uncommon and provides an example of the types of pressure placed on individuals with reproductive problems.)

Some couples set limits of time and/or extent of infertility investigation and treatment. For example, a 38-year-old may agree to all hormonal investigations and minor procedures, including laparoscopy and operative endoscopy, but will stop treatment if major surgery is indicated. Alternatively, a 39-year-old may set a time deadline, stating she will cease treatment on her 40th birthday. Such deadlines are generally unhealthy since they create additional, unnecessary (because they are self-imposed) pressures.

Ending Active Treatment and Considering Adoption

Regardless of the reason, once couples have decided to cease active treatment, they may choose a life without children or consider adoption. In either event, these couples should be aware that conception, though unlikely, may occur later. Such conceptions are common in those with:

- Patent tubes
- Oligoasthenospermia

Pregnancy or no pregnancy, once adoption has been considered, the couple must individually and mutually find the concept acceptable if it is to be successful. At this point, counseling and physician, family and group support is extremely important.

Adoption must be a positive and active decision rather than an anticipated stop-gap to save a failing marriage; the latter could have negative consequences on an adoptive child. To avoid this situation, most adoption institutions request an investigation of a couple's medical, psychological and marital status during the screening of both parties as acceptable candidates for adoption. Included in screening are such questions as:

- Is each partner physically healthy and anticipated to have a normal life expectancy?
- Are partners psychologically stable and mature?
- Will the couple make loving parents for the baby?
- Is this a stable, warm, loving household. Is the marital environment considered a positive one for the child?
- Is the couple capable of providing for the child in a reasonable material fashion?

Such screening has serious medical and ethical connotations. It is considered of paramount importance that, just as a positive and stable marriage should have the privilege of attaining a child, a baby should be assured of living in a loving and stable home which can provide for its emotional, spiritual and materialistic needs.

Institutional vs. Private Adoption Services

Many agencies often related to religious institutions provide adoption services to their communities, and some couples pursue adoption through these parties. Other couples pursue private adoptions, usually completed by reputable, registered attorneys. Assistance in finding local institutional or legal assistance for adoption may be obtained by contacting local RESOLVE chapters or infertility specialists. To obtain further information, write: RESOLVE, Inc.; 5 Water Street; Arlington, MA 02174-4814.

Closed vs. Open Adoption

Closed Adoption

In closed adoption, a child is placed with a couple in an anonymous manner. The natural mother neither knows nor meets the couple to whom her child has been given, and the couple is unaware of the identity of the baby's mother. This situation is probably the healthiest, reflecting the ultimate decision of the natural mother to part with her baby as a final one.

Even in closed adoption, if the natural mother does not part with her baby at birth (some do not), she may change her mind and want to keep her baby. If this should occur, the canceled adoption is far less devastating to the adoptive parents than if it were to occur months or years later as can occur in open adoption.

Usually the couple receives the baby within days or weeks of the baby's being given up (often soon after birth). The natural mother then may resume her life pursuits, and she and the adoptive parents are free to reap the positive rewards of their mutual decisions.

In closed adoption, the adoptive couple is far more secure about the circumstances of adoption. The new parents feel more secure that the natural mother is less likely to regret her decision and are, thus, freed from days and weeks of decision-making and possible harassment by the natural mother, as can happen when the status is open.

Open Adoption

In open adoption, the adoptive parents are aware of the identity of the natural mother (even during her pregnancy), and the natural mother knows the couple with whom her baby has been placed. These circumstances are far more conducive to later visitations between the natural mother and child and can lead to possible questions and challenges regarding visitation rights, the original adoption and the possible appeal for return of the baby to the natural mother. At the very least, such challenges can lead to changes in the date that a baby is given to the adoptive parents, which can cause major disappointments to an already anxious, anticipatory couple.

Such disasters and potentially tragic circumstances can and must be avoided through adequate counseling and screening of both parties prior to their entering into adoption agreements. All parties involved should be assisted and supported emotionally by physicians, counselors, families, friends and support groups during this trying period, and the support must never waiver until all legal and fiscal pursuits are completed and the new baby is safely and finally placed.

A new baby in the home is truly a time for celebration. Commonly, adoptive parents send announcement cards and host parties for the new child in order to assure that all involved will accept and recognize the child as the couple's own. Though the decision to adopt is, itself, a major psychological and emotional relief, the arrival of the baby greatly reinforces these positive emotions. Additionally, partners who are relieved of the demanding infertility diagnostic and treatment schedules are likely to experience a better quality of life.

Most couples find the cessation of active treatment, the resumption of normal life and the challenges of becoming new parents to be very positive times. Their reproductive needs, most commonly, have been positively fulfilled by their decision to become adoptive parents and their acting upon that decision.

Occasionally, one partner may rekindle the need for "another try" at conception. If new treatment options are available, clinicians should counsel patients about them and assist with subsequent treatment. If, however, the decision to adopt was made because of irreversible, untreatable infertility, the couple should be fully reminded, informed, counseled and supported accordingly through their period of indecision.

Overall, adoption should be reviewed as an option for every couple from the earliest stages of investigation of infertility and whenever couples seek further knowledge about or assistance with this option. Couples interested in adoption should be triaged to reputable institutions or legal sources who are equipped to advise and assist them with this option.

#27 Operative Endoscopy

Introduction

Major advancements in gynecological endoscopy have occurred in this past decade. Improved optic, fiberoptic and fluid light conduction systems have facilitated better diagnostic and therapeutic capabilities in the field of reproductive surgery. The role of operative endoscopy within the context of the investigation and treatment of infertility is outlined in Figure 27.1.

Current common procedures for the diagnosis and treatment and/or correction of infertility are hysteroscopy and laparoscopy. Surgical instruments and laser systems facilitate the clinicians' abilities to correct minor and, sometimes, relatively major anatomical abnormalities via the hysteroscope/laparoscope. These operations constitute the field of gynecological endoscopy (pelviscopy).

Procedures performed via the hysteroscope include:

- Transection of uterine septa
- Division of intrauterine synechiae
- Removal of intrauterine polyps
- Resection of submucous myomas
- Cannulation, dilatation, and/or removal of cornual/isthmic tubal occlusions (catheter/balloon tuboplasty)

Procedures performed via the laparoscope include:

- Lysis of adhesions
- Coagulation/vaporization of pelvic endometriosis
- Salpingolysis
- Ovariolysis
- Drainage and vaporization of ovarian cysts/endometriomas
- Removal of ovarian cysts/endometriomas
- Drainage of multiple follicles in polycystic ovarian syndrome
- Drainage, coagulation, vaporization and/or excision of congenital cysts of epoöphoron or paroöphoron

- Transection and removal of hydatid cysts of Morgagni
- Biopsies of lesions of the:
  - Peritoneum
  - Fallopian tubes
  - Ovaries
- Irrigation and cell block of peritoneal washings
- Chromopertubation and pelvic irrigation
- Drainage of pelvic abscesses and/or pyosalpinges
- Fimbrioplasty/salpingoneostomy
- Salpingotomy for evacuation of products of conception in ectopic pregnancy with:
  - Tubal conservation OR
  - Laparoscopic resection of partial or total oviduct

Instrumentation

New instrumentation for these surgical advances includes:

- Verres needles, reusable or disposable
- Trocar and cannula:
  - Reusable or disposable
  - Pyramidal or conical
- Laparoscopes:
  - Diagnostic (5 to 10 mm)
  - Operative (8 to 12 mm)

The main cannula should be non-insulated to facilitate electrical conduction to the periumbilical skin in the event of capacitance of electrical energy within the pelvis; this is preferable to short circuit of electrical energy to a nearby structure (eg, bowel).

The second-puncture and other cannula include:

- 5 mm Insulated cannulas for working with coagulators
- Metallic cannulas with lasers

Conical trocars (which are less likely to transect blood vessels than other trocars) are used for multiple punctures after the anterior abdominal wall vasculature has been illuminated and defined by the laparoscope.

Conical trocars are always inserted under direct vision within the peritoneal cavity, while observing subperitoneal blood vessels via the main laparoscope. This technique facilitates the safe entry of additional probes and instruments into the abdomen.

Most major operative techniques involve double-puncture methods. The double-channel technique allows surgery to be performed via a large panoramic view from the main observing channel to facilitate command of the operative field; procedures are then completed from additional channels.

The double-channel method precludes the sudden appearance of the bowel or other structure into the operative field, as can occur in single-puncture operative methods, though the single-channel operating laparoscope is preferred in certain circumstances because it offers easy visualization and access to pathology directly in front of the laparoscope.

Second-puncture instruments include:

- Probes (centimeter scale)
- Suction cannula
- Suction and irrigation cannula
- Irrigation cannula
- Scissors
- Needles
- Knives
- Bipolar button electrode and irrigation channel
- Bipolar grasping forceps
- Unipolar grasping forceps
- Unipolar button electrode, with or without irrigation channels (electrocoagulation uses non-electrolyte solutions)
- Endotherm:
  - Button
  - Knife
  - Grasping probes
  - Grasping forceps
- Mobilizing platform instruments
- CO_2 laser operating laparoscope
- Second probe, with or without backstops (necessary for CO_2 laser safety)

- Non-reflective probes and backstops for CO_2 laser surgery
- Fiberoptic laser conduction channels, with or without suction irrigation, for such laser systems as:
  - Argon
  - KTP-532
  - Sapphire-tipped YAG

Common operative methods involve either:

- Watching through the main channel and using two additional channels for:
  - Grasping
  - Cutting or vaporizing, OR
- Grasping through the second puncture and operating with the operating laparoscope via the main puncture site

Principles of Laser Safety

Principles which must be maintained for the safe use of laser equipment are that:

- The laser technician maintains command and control of the laser
- The operating room door has a sign reading "Laser In Use"
- The operating room windows are covered by appropriate shutters
- The patient's eyes are closed and protected by wet pads (CO_2) or appropriate glasses
- Lasers used include:
  - YAG
  - Argon
  - KTP-532
  - CO_2
- All staff wear appropriate, wave-length protective glasses
- The patient's abdomen is flooded with irrigation fluid (CO_2)
- The laser is always set on "Standby" when not in use by the surgeon or when the surgeon hesitates during a procedure

- The foot pedal is specifically placed, to avoid its possible confusion with the electrocoagulator pedal
- The communication of commands and responses (ie, "Laser On" and "Standby") between the surgeon and laser technician are clearly spoken and repeated to one another to avoid confusion and to minimize the margin for error
- The surgeon clarifies his/her choices of laser wattage and pulse before beginning vaporization and after every significant pause during the procedure

Scheduling and Organization of the Operating Room

Surgery staff must be specifically trained in operative laparoscopy and endoscopy and be aware of and repeatedly in-service trained for preparation and care of laparoscopic and endoscopic instrumentation. The staff must be trained and knowledgeable in the use of insufflators, coagulators and laser systems.

Organization and scheduling of the operating room, especially in major hospitals with large gynecological staffs, are greatly affected by diagnostic and operative laparoscopy, which usually require 30 minutes to one hour and one and one-half to two hours, respectively. Adequately-staffed and equipped, specialized, operative endoscopy suites have been established both with and without laser facilities.

Though specialized equipment must be readily available, many surgical cases do not require all instruments and/or laser use; the percentage of non-use is relatively high and must be anticipated 20 to 40 percent of the time.

Physicians must specifically book "operative endoscopy" and request an estimated two and one-half hours for the procedure if an orderly flow of patients through the operating room is to be maintained.

Preoperative Counseling and Consent

Patients should be advised regarding operative endoscopy and should be made aware of the risks of laparotomy.

The three major outcomes at surgery are:

- Simple diagnostic laparoscopy – For no significant pathology
- Operative endoscopy (pelviscopy) – For mild to moderate pathology which will respond to operative laparoscopy
- Laparotomy – For severe and/or extensive disease or for pathology which is adjacent to major blood vessels, the bowel or the ureter

  In cases with extensive pathology:

  - The extent of the disease is documented
  - Patients are counseled regarding findings and alternative therapies, including:
    - Microsurgical pelvic reconstruction
    - IVF or GIFT
    - Consideration of adoption

Operative Principles

All patients must be proven to be chlamydia culture negative prior to surgery, and most patients are given prophylactic antibiotics (usually cephalosporins), perioperatively.

During the procedure, an insufflator with automatic (pressure to +14 mm Hg) and manual (pressure as high as 50 mm Hg) manometer pressure gauges is used to minimize the risks associated with Verres needles and to aid control of insufflation pressures.

For prolonged procedures, it is essential that the patient's cardiovascular status be adequately monitored; this is done through EKGs and the monitoring of vital signs, CO_2 and PO_2.

For the procedure, the abdomen is safely insufflated, and the laparoscopic trocar and cannula are inserted. After the anterior abdominal vasculature is defined, additional punctures are completed with conical trocars in relative darkness, while carefully avoiding the blood vessels which are under direct vision through the laparoscope.

The need to remove smoke plume necessitates the timely refill of the abdomen by "manual" or "fast flow" insufflators. These are monitored and carefully controlled by the circulating nurse who specifically ensures that intra-abdominal pressures never rise above 14 (preferable) to 18 mm Hg.

If hemostasis or hydrodissection is required, intermittent peritoneal irrigation is performed via the irrigating channel, using Ringer's lactate (unless an electrical current with electrolyte-free, five-percent dextrose is used). The Ringer's lactate is poured through the irrigator at pressures of 120 to 200 mm Hg and is suctioned via the suction cannula, which has multiple holes to prevent traction injuries to adjacent pelvic organs. The Ringer's lactate irrigation is heparinized with 2,000 IU heparin/L and includes ampicillin 100 mg/L (may be replaced by erythromycin in penicillin-sensitive patients) and corticosteroid 100 mg/L.

In accordance with general microsurgical principles, 200 mL of the irrigation solution and/or 50 mL dextran 70 is left in the pelvis after the procedure is completed. (The risks of allergy to dextran must always be borne in mind; some surgeons prefer the Ringer's/corticosteroid solution.)

Postoperative Expectations and Care

After surgery, patients:

- Are usually discharged within six to 12 hours
- Are to be relatively non-ambulatory for 48 hours
- Should leave their surgical wounds, closed primarily with subcutaneous and subcuticular absorbable sutures, covered with steri-strips and Band-Aids for five to seven days
- Are to take oral analgesics
- Will experience some shoulder or neck pain, from residual gas of pneumoperitoneum, for 24 to 48 hours
- Will experience some burning on micturition, from catheter insertion, for 24 to 48 hours
- Will experience vaginal loss for three to four days
- Will resume regular bladder and bowel functions within two to three days

- Should experience no fever greater than 99 degrees F
- Are to keep wounds dry for five to seven days, after which steri-strips or Band-Aids may be removed
- May resume regular activities within three to four days
- May resume sexual activity after three to four days or two days after cessation of blood flow if post-operative vaginal bleeding has occurred

At postoperative follow-up visit, patients are to be counseled regarding:

- The overall procedure
- Diagnostic photographs
- The operative outcome diagnosis
- Therapeutic options
- Plans for further therapy

TABLE 27.1 – **Principles of Surgical Management for Patients With Reproductive Disorders**

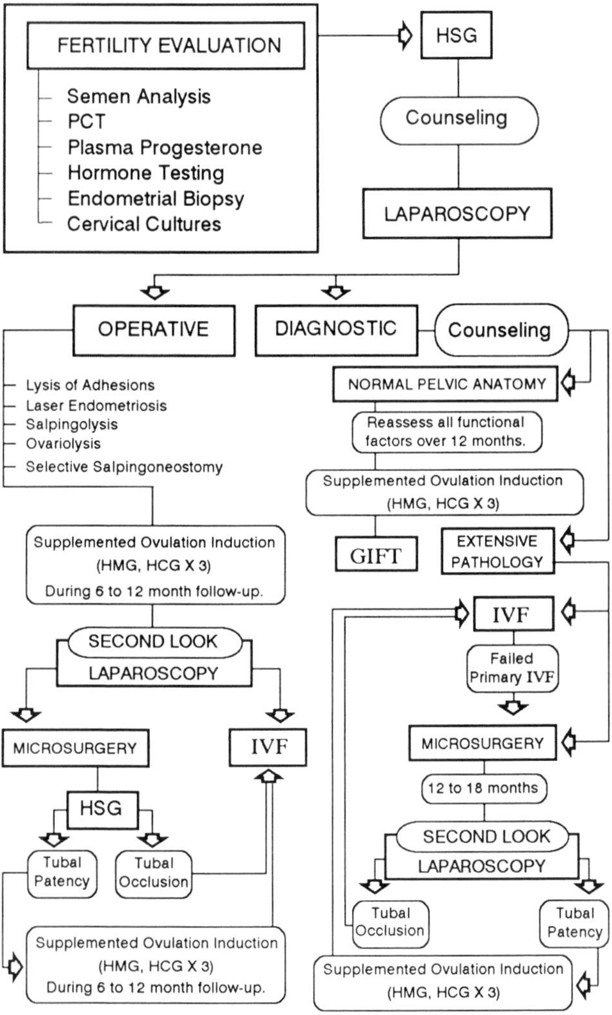

Reproduced with permission of the Fertility Center of North Texas, Dallas, Texas, 1991.

NOTES

#28 Sperm Enhancement Techniques

Introduction

The advent of assisted reproductive technology (ART) and the accomplishment of successful *in vitro* fertilization (IVF) heralded a new era as it demonstrated that sperm may be rendered capable of fertilizing ova in an artificial environment.

Under normal physiologic conditions, ejaculate is deposited into the vagina, and healthy sperm traverse the female genital tract toward mature ova. The cervical mucus plays a major role in the selection of healthy sperm, which become further capacitated within the endometrial cavity and oviduct fluids. Fertilization of an ovum by an activated spermatozoa usually takes place in the outer ampulla of the fallopian tube.

The direct deposit of semen into the uterine cavity is contraindicated because of the risk of introducing infection or foreign antigenic substances possibly present in seminal plasma. However, sperm can be separated from its seminal plasma and deposited into the uterus, an attractive option for selected couples with cervical factors and/or male oligospermic/asthenospermic dysfunctions.

Additionally, technological methods of enhancing sperm function range from simple to highly complex and include such specific treatments for specific causes of infertility as:

- Active antibiotic therapy for pyospermia
- HMG therapy for hypogonadotropic hypogonadism
- Split ejaculate for hypervolemia (see Section #10)
- Mechanically breaking up thickened, clumped sperm through a 20-gauge needle in non-liquefying semen samples
- Washed sperm intrauterine insemination (WIUI)

Washed Sperm Intrauterine Insemination

Washed sperm intrauterine insemination (WIUI) is the most common sperm enhancement technique currently in use. It involves:

- The washing and immediate insemination of sperm
- The post-wash "swim up" technique
- The passage of washed sperm through various gradients, eg, hyaluronidase, sperm select or Percoll®
- The use of previously washed and/or incubated sperm for IVF
- Assisting sperm function by physically treating the cumulus, zona or ovum, eg:
  - Cumulus stripping
  - Partial zona removal
  - Zona drilling techniques

Artificial Insemination (Including WIUI)

Some authorities prefer WIUI to the standard insemination techniques of depositing sperm in the cervical mucus or of using a cervical cup. Indications for insemination which include WIUI are:

- Male factors of:
  - Oligospermia
  - Asthenospermia
  - Moderate levels of antisperm antibodies
  - Situational impotence
  - Low sperm volumes
- Female cervical factors of:
  - Stenosis
  - Previous cautery, laser vaporization or cryotherapy
  - Previous cone biopsy with excision of cervical glands
  - Repeatedly poor cervical mucus
  - Repeatedly poor postcoital tests after specific correction of cervical and male factors, eg:
    - Chronic infected cervical erosion even with adequate antibiotic therapy
    - Oligoasthenospermia in absence of general or specific male factors

Method of Sperm Preparation

Sperm is collected by masturbation or partner manipulation. The original ejaculate may be submitted as a single sample or as a split ejaculate when volumes are greater than 5 mL (see Section #10). If sperm antibodies are present, the sperm may be placed directly into the culture medium.

The ejaculate is placed in a sterile tube, and all apparatus and equipment are kept in an incubator at 37 degrees C (body temperature) and an atmosphere of five-percent CO_2 in air. The culture medium may vary, but a common medium is sterile Ham's F-10 prewarmed to 37 degrees C. This medium may be supplemented by 10 percent of the female partner's serum, drawn during the periovulatory period, provided she has no antisperm antibodies.

Laboratory Technique

The ejaculate is diluted with 3 to 5 mL of the culture medium in a centrifuge tube which has been sealed with sterile paraffin paper. It is placed on an agitator, where it is shaken for one minute. Next, the test tube is placed in the centrifuge and spun at 3,000 rpm for three minutes. The tube is then withdrawn, its paraffin paper cover removed, and the supernatant poured out, leaving a sperm pellet at the bottom of the centrifuge tube.

Two mL of culture medium are added to the tube, which is then resealed, agitated and centrifuged. The supernatant is discarded a second time, following which 1.5 mL of the tissue culture medium is added to the sperm pellet.

The technologist has two options at this point in the procedure:

- The sperm may be agitated within the culture medium and left to stand for 30 minutes to three hours so that debris will fall to the bottom of the test tube and the remaining spermatozoa in the supernatant aspirated for intrauterine insemination OR

- The swim up technique in which the pellet may be left at the base of the test tube and incubated for one to four hours to allow viable sperm actively to swim up from the pellet into the supernatant fluid

In either case, the supernatant containing sperm is then drawn into a 1 cc sterile tuberculin syringe, loaded into a sterile catheter and transferred into the uterine cavity via the cervix (Figure 28.1).

Insemination

Insemination is performed after confirmation that ovulation is imminent. This is done by an LH surge guide and/or an ultrasound assessment of the dominant follicle at 36 hours post-HCG injection.

Clinical Procedure

To perform insemination, the physician is to:

- Place the patient in the lithotomy position
- Insert a speculum into the vagina
- Cleanse the cervix with a clean cotton bud
- Gently apply a tenaculum, and pass a sterile transfer catheter into the uterus
- Gently insert the washed sperm sample into the uterine cavity
- Withdraw the catheter and tenaculum
- Remove the speculum
- Instruct the patient to lie on the examining couch for approximately 10 minutes

A most important consideration of insemination is that washed sperm do not have the longevity (ie, 24 to 48 hours) of sperm spontaneously ejaculated into healthy cervical mucus. It is assumed that washed sperm live only 8 to 12 hours, implying that the timing of insemination to ovulation is essential if WIUI is to be successful.

Some authorities recommend postponing insemination until confirmation of LH surge and of rupture of the dominant ovarian follicle. This delay is in the hope that ovum pickup by the tubal fimbriae has occurred and that the ovum has moved to the oviduct and is ready for fertilization.

Clinicians also recommend transperitoneal insemination using a sterile technique via the cul-de-sac, but little data exist to reliably comment on the merit of this technique.

Irrespective of the method used, all health care providers should be concerned about and diligent to time WIUI as closely as possible to the time of predicted ovulation. In practical terms, it is common for patients to be given 5,000 to 10,000 units of HCG at the appropriate time in the menstrual cycle and insemination to follow 34 to 36 hours later.

Number of Inseminations and Anticipated Results

For good results, WIUI should be performed for three to six cycles. The expectation is that correctly-selected patients will achieve gestation at some time during these inseminations. The incidence of pregnancy per cycle for the WIUI technique is approximately:

- Five to seven percent when completed in spontaneous cycles
- 10 to 14 percent when completed in clomiphene-stimulated cycles
- 18 to 21 percent when completed in HMG- and HCG-administered cycles

The varying percentages may well reflect subtle ovulatory dysfunctions and the need for their correction, as well as the need to precisely time insemination in order to optimize chances of conception. WIUI techniques have resulted in many pregnancies, but further data must be accumulated for more specific guidelines regarding their widespread use.

Isolated cases of possible acquisition of antisperm antibodies in females subjected to multiple courses of WIUI have been reported. Until these data can be confirmed or denied, it is imperative that WIUI be reserved for selected patients who have abnormal post-coital tests and abnormal cervical and/or sperm function and that the technique not be used on a purely empiric basis.

Since the WIUI procedure involves passing sperm directly through the cervical canal, this method may be of particular value for women with an abnormal cervical factor due to:

- Previous freezing
- Cauterization
- Radical cone biopsy

The procedure is also the treatment of choice for men with causes of infertility relating to sperm, such as:

- Oligospermia
- Asthenospermia
- Low volume with low normal numbers
- Sperm antibodies in the semen but not the washed spermatozoa

WIUI is a simple office procedure which facilitates the preparation of sperm for transfer into the uterine cavity. It appears to be helpful in the oligospermic male refractory to other modalities of treatment (hormonal or surgical) and has played a major role in the preparation and capacitation of sperm for GIFT and IVF.

Additional Sperm Preparation Techniques

Much research and data is being generated about additional sperm preparation techniques. Currently studied are the techniques of passing sperm through various columns of isotonic agents and of preparations using albumin, Ethiodol®, Percoll® and/or Sephadex® layers at the base of the centrifuge tube. These techniques are thought to improve sperm quality and motility and to enable the isolation and selection of X- or Y-bearing sperm (to influence the sex of the conceptus).

(For further information, see Section #10, Semen Analysis; Section #12, Postcoital Test; Section #13, Hormonal Testing: Male; Section #18, Male Factor; Section #19, Abnormal Postcoital Test; and Section #24, Immunological Infertility.)

FIGURE 28.1 — **Preparation of Sperm for Washed Intrauterine Insemination**

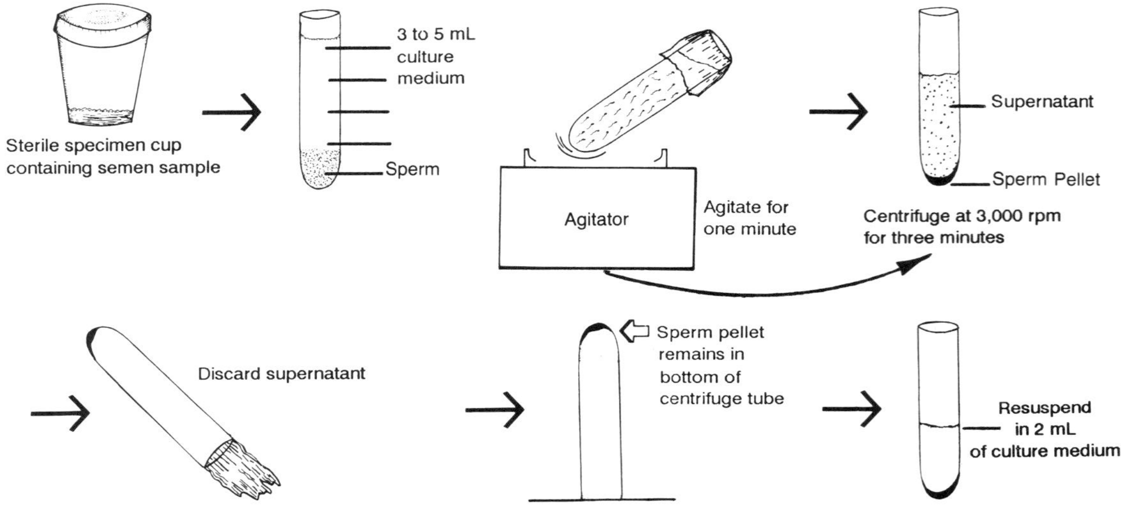

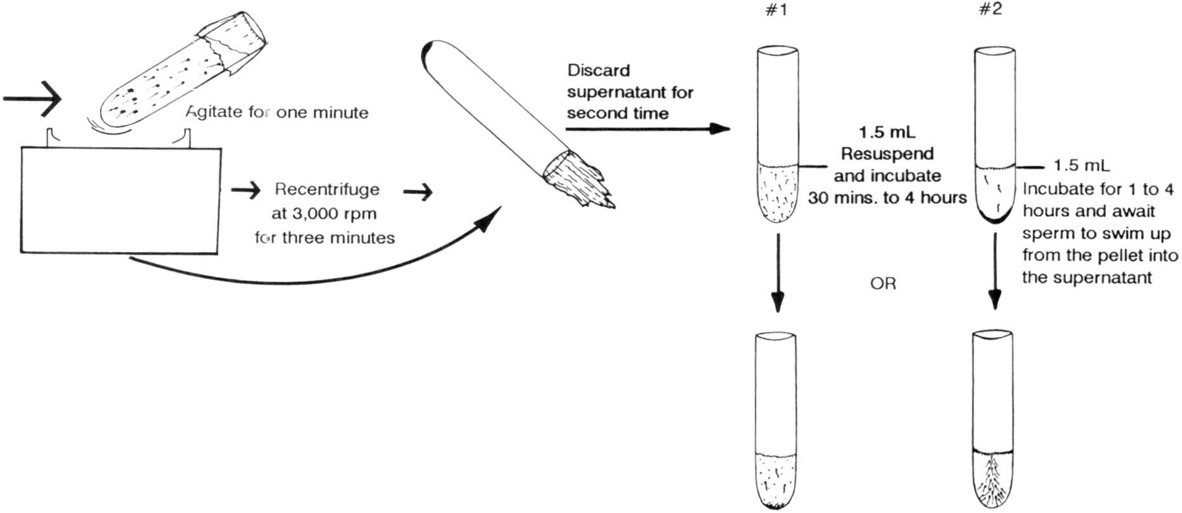

Agitate for one minute
Recentrifuge at 3,000 rpm for three minutes
Discard supernatant for second time
#1
1.5 mL
Resuspend and incubate 30 mins. to 4 hours
OR
#2
1.5 mL
Incubate for 1 to 4 hours and await sperm to swim up from the pellet into the supernatant

#29 Gamete Intrafallopian Transfer (GIFT)

Introduction

In the gamete intrafallopian transfer (GIFT) method, ova are aspirated from the surface of the ovary and placed together with prepared sperm in the distal tubal ampulla. Theoretically, if fertilization occurs, the cleaving morula is retained in the oviduct's ampulla until its timely discharge into the uterine cavity via the proximal oviduct.

The constituents of tubal fluid provide the ideal environment which facilitates fertilization, early cleavage of the morula and its development into a blastocyst. It is not surprising, then, that ova and sperm placed together in the tubal environment will result in pregnancy in a significant number of cases. GIFT has been followed by success rates of 20 to 40 percent.

Goals and Objectives

The goals and objectives of the GIFT procedure are to:

- Obtain multiple mature ova
- Combine ova with prepared and capacitated sperm
- Place combined ova and sperm in the ampulla of the oviducts

Instrumentation and Operative Techniques

Couples desiring conception via the GIFT procedure must have undergone simpler treatments, including supplemented ovulation induction with HMG and washed sperm intrauterine insemination (WIUI), before considering GIFT. Additionally, patients selected for the procedure must have healthy, patent oviducts.

Prior to the GIFT procedure, patients are stimulated to produce multiple ova through the use of:

- Clomiphene citrate plus HMG plus HCG
- HMG plus HCG
- Pure FSH, HMG and HCG
- HMG plus GnRH agonists with HCG

Plasma estradiol and urinary or plasma LH are monitored daily once estradiol levels begin to rise. Pelvic ultrasounds are performed on alternate days and then daily as significant estradiol elevations occur.

Both ovaries are visualized, and all visible follicles greater than 10 mm in diameter are documented. If and when more than five follicles greater than 16 to 18 mm appear in the absence of a spontaneous LH surge, an injection of HCG 5,000 to 10,000 IU is given, and patients are prepared for laparoscopy and GIFT. The procedure should be performed 34 hours after HCG administration.

Four to six hours before the operation, sperm is collected, washed and preincubated in the laboratory.

During laparoscopy, the uterus is manipulated as little as possible. For laparoscopic insertion, the abdomen is insufflated with CO_2. Once safe insertion of the pneumoperitoneum is accomplished, many GIFT surgeons wash the CO_2 out of the peritoneum and replace it with a mixture of N_2O or air (90 percent), O_2 (five percent) and CO_2 (five percent). (Exchange of the gases is done in an effort to reduce the incidence of hypercarbia and acidemia which has potential negative effects on ova in the follicles and may acidify the tissue culture medium.)

A 12- to 16-gauge needle is then inserted through a second puncture site. The needle is used to penetrate each follicle, while the ovary is held steady with atraumatic grasping forceps which have been passed through a third puncture site (Figure 16.4).

The follicular fluid is collected at a pressure of approximately 100 mm Hg, and the follicle is either washed out with a double-puncture needle or the same needle is flushed in and out with culture medium until bloodstaining from the follicle is encountered. The follicle is filled and emptied a few times, and the fluid is transferred to the laboratory adjacent to the operating room.

In the laboratory, each test tube of follicular contents is labeled separately and examined under a dissection microscope to confirm the presence or absence of ova in the fluid. Each ovum is graded on a scale of one to five and classified as immature or mature.

Ova graded as mature (four to five) are considered healthy and likely to be successfully fertilized. Two to three of these ova are loaded, together with 50,000 to 100,000 prepared and capacitated sperm, in an inert, sterile, transfer catheter, which is immediately passed back to the operating room. The catheter is inserted into the distal end of the oviduct about 2 to 3 cm into the ampulla, where the gametes are released. Usually, two to three ova are transferred into each fallopian tube.

The catheter is then returned to the laboratory for confirmation that no ova are present in the catheter and that they have been successfully transferred into the oviducts.

After hemostasis in the pelvis is confirmed, all gas is exsufflated from the abdomen and abdominal wounds are sutured, using non-reactive, absorbable sutures.

The patient is given an injection of 25 mg progesterone in oil IM and is discharged six to 12 hours later. Progesterone injections (25 mg) are continued daily.

The patient is to be ambulatory but relatively quiescent for 48 to 72 hours, after which she may resume her normal activities. Plasma βHCG is drawn 10 to 12 days later and is repeated in 48 hours to confirm the presence or absence of pregnancy. If βHCG rises, progesterone supplementation is continued and early ultrasound is completed at about six weeks to confirm clinical gestation and to rule out possible ectopic pregnancy.

Theoretical Advantage

The GIFT method assumes that the major defect has been failure of ovum pickup and that placing ova and sperm in the natural physiological site (the oviduct) will accomplish conception.

Disadvantage

The disadvantage of GIFT is the inability to observe fertilization and cleavage of embryos. This means that in unsuccessful attempts, patients have no way of determining if fertilization failure was the reason for failure of conception.

Results

Successful clinical pregnancy and live births have occurred in 20 to 40 percent of patients undergoing the GIFT procedure. The highest success rate has generally been observed for couples who have been diagnosed with idiopathic infertility in whom the female partner is normal and the male partner has normal seminal parameters.

GIFT has also been successful for couples in whom attempts at conception by donor insemination has failed. However, if the male partner's seminal parameters are markedly abnormal (eg, severe oligospermia [less than 10 million] or asthenospermia), success rates are significantly lower.

GIFT is a highly positive technique offered to patients who have healthy oviducts and in whom prior methods of fertility treatment (including three cycles of supplemented ovulation induction with HMG, HCG and progesterone therapy) have failed.

#30 In Vitro Fertilization (IVF)

Goals and Objectives

The goals of *in vitro* fertilization (IVF) are:

- Fertilization of the ovum, with subsequent cleavage
- Return of the embryo into the uterine cavity, followed by implantation and normal gestation

These objectives have been achieved in the experimental animal for many years, but it was not until the birth of Louise Brown, a baby conceived *in vitro* by Steptoe and Edwards in 1978, that the technique showed promise for application in human females. In the past 10 years, a few thousand babies have been born following use of this method.

Basic Principles

In IVF, mature ova are harvested from their follicles by transvaginal retrieval under ultrasound monitoring or at laparoscopy. Semen is prepared in culture media which enhance the sperm's capacity for ovum penetration.

The harvested ova and sperm are cultured in a Petri dish in a meticulously quality-controlled incubator environment in which fertilized ova cleave into healthy blastomeres. Selected four- to eight-cell embryos are loaded into a catheter and passed through the cervical canal into the uterine cavity approximately 36 to 48 hours after fertilization. If implantation occurs, measurement of plasma βHCG is possible approximately 10 days later.

Steptoe and Edwards' initial success resulted from harvesting a single ovum in a natural cycle, but subsequent data have indicated improved success rates with hyperstimulation of the female and the harvesting of multiple follicles.

The incidence of pregnancy has been highest when three to six embryos are transferred, but this is also associated with a higher incidence of multiple pregnancies, including triplets and quadruplets, with high abortion rates or significant problems of prematurity and perinatal mortality. Ideally, at least three embryos should be transferred.

Cryopreservation of extra embryos facilitates an opportunity for patients to return for IVF during natural cycles so that embryo transfer can occur under "normal" physiological conditions. This concept and technique has met with early success, but preliminary results have been disappointing. Again, success requires the transfer of at least two to three embryos.

Principles of Stimulation Protocols

Stimulation protocols have included the use of:

- Clomiphene citrate, followed by HMG and HCG
- HMG plus pure FSH, followed by HCG

The associated use of GnRH agonists with down regulation of the pituitary has facilitated far more control of ovarian hyperstimulation techniques and has minimized the incidence of cancellation due to:

- Premature LH surges OR
- The inability to achieve abundant mature follicles at the appropriate time of the menstrual cycle

Controlled ovarian hyperstimulation with resultant harvesting of multiple mature follicles may facilitate transfer of two to three embryos in the initial cycle, together with the patient returning for at least two further transfers of cryopreserved embryos during the same year.

With this protocol, some Australian workers have projected an expectation of pregnancy in 40 to 50 percent of patients as the result of two major harvestings and four cryopreserved embryo transfers in a single year.

Case Selection

Because the overall success rate for IVF (live births per treatment cycle) is between 10 and 15 percent per cycle, this technique is reserved for those in whom prior and more simplified methods of conception have failed.

Common indications for IVF include:

- Absence of oviducts due to:
  - Pelvic inflammatory disease (PID) OR
  - Tubal excision following ectopic gestation
- Failure of previous medical and surgical therapy for endometriosis
- Idiopathic infertility in which all prior techniques have failed (including three cycles of supplemented ovulation induction with HMG)
- Inadequate male factor
- The presence of antisperm antibodies in the female in which IVF can be accomplished in the presence of antibody-free donor serum
- The presence of male antisperm antibodies

Conditions to be fulfilled to qualify for IVF include:

- Couples with psychological and marital stability who have been adequately counseled regarding methods of stimulation and fertilization yet who are fully aware of a potentially negative outcome when confronted with success rates of 20 to 25 percent per transfer cycle
- The presence of a healthy uterine cavity and relative ease of access through the cervical canal
- Proven adequacy of the endometrium in prior stimulation, with confirmed adequate "in-phase" endometrial biopsy and known length of uterine cavity
- Absence of cervical and/or uterine (pelvic) infection, including:
  - Chlamydia
  - Mycoplasma
  - Ureaplasma
- Absence of and/or prior treatment for:
  - Hyperprolactinemia
  - Thyroid dysfunction
  - Hyperandrogenism
- Known gonadotropin status (ie, FSH:LH ratios)
- Prior assessment of ovulation induction response or evidence of adequate residual ovarian function, particularly in patients who have had repeated and extensive ovarian resection surgery

- Thorough evaluation of male and previous screening and semen analysis to exclude seminal infection
- Adequacy of numbers regarding normal morphology and motility, together with exclusion of excessive auto-antibodies
- Prior normal hamster penetration test with a penetration rate greater than 10 percent

Principles of Management

Patient Counseling

It is essential that couples be fully aware of the facts that:

- The treatment cycle may not be completed, due to:
  - Inadequate stimulation of an adequate number of mature follicles
  - The occurrence of a premature LH surge
- Despite proceeding to egg retrieval, fertilization may not occur
- Despite fertilization and assessed timely transfer of adequate healthy embryos, pregnancy will not occur in 75 to 80 percent of attempts
- Pregnancy will be confirmed at a timely ultrasound to exclude chemical pregnancy or blighted ovum. Patients' prior knowledge and understanding of this possibility will avoid much dismay and depression if gestation is found to be non-viable
- When more than three embryos are transferred, the incidence of multiple pregnancy, including triplets and quadruplets, is significant (this may present obstetric and prenatal problems)
- The option of:
  - Discarding excess embryos
  - Cryopreserving excess embryos and returning for future embryo transfer

Such factors imply in-depth psychological screening and counseling of couples seeking IVF, since the success rate per cycle is no higher than 10 to 15 percent, despite positive motivation, cost and effort. If embryo transfer is completed, the rate increases only to 20 to 25 percent. These facts must be clearly understood by all participating couples.

On the positive side, clinicians should encourage couples to attempt at least two to three IVF procedures, because the cumulative chance of achieving pregnancy is as high as 40 to 50 percent with multiple attempts.

A Treatment Cycle

Ovulation induction of multiple ova for harvesting at mid-cycle is accomplished by:

- Clomiphene citrate at 100 mg daily for five days, followed by HMG at 150 IU daily thereafter
- HMG at two to four ampules per day from the second to third day of the menstrual cycle
- Pure FSH from the second day of the menstrual cycle for two to four days, together with HMG, which is continued until ovulation induction
- Combinations of the above

Recent reports have indicated a significantly higher success rate with GnRH therapy in selected cases (see *Recent Innovations* below), and many groups have shown that a more predictable cycle with a lower incidence of cancellation of cycles can be accomplished by the administration of GnRH agonists prior to ovulation induction. The GnRH agonist, given during the secretory/luteal phase of the previous cycle, shuts down the secretion of pituitary-gonadotropins so that ovulation induction stimulation with HMG is completed without the risk of a premature LH surge. Patients using GnRH agonist therapy require larger doses of gonadotropins.

In some institutions, measurements of FSH:LH ratios at the onset of menses and documentation of GnRH agonist, gonadotropin and estradiol responses assist in planning therapy for ovulation induction in individual cycles. The objective of ovulation induction is to provide multiple healthy and mature follicles for harvesting. A premature LH surge and/or inadequate numbers of follicles cancel the harvest cycle.

Harvesting of Ova

If multiple follicles are observed and many are greater than 16 mm in diameter, HCG is given and ovum collection can be carried out approximately 36 hours later. Ovum collection may be completed either transvaginally with ultrasound monitoring using a vaginal probe or at laparoscopy.

Vaginal retrieval, a far less invasive technique than laparoscopy, is highly acceptable, and comparable pregnancy rates have made it the method of choice. The procedure is performed in an operating or sterile room.

To perform the procedure:

- The patient is given light sedation and is provided adequate anesthetic monitoring
- Local anesthesia is administered in the form of vaginal and paracervical low-dosage dilute lignocaine
- The vagina is thoroughly prepared and irrigated with:
  - Ringer's lactate OR
  - Saline OR
  - Tissue culture medium
- Under transvaginal ultrasound guidance, the ovary is entered with a 16-gauge needle and stabbed a minimal number of times to achieve the maximal retrieval of follicles
- The aspiration needle may be irrigated and repeatedly removed or a double-channel needle may be used to facilitate flushing and aspiration
- Follicular fluid in the collection chamber is immediately submitted to the embryologist in an adjacent laboratory for confirmation of ova presence
- Once ovum retrieval is confirmed, the surgeon aspirates and evacuates as many subsequent follicles as possible
- The patient is discharged within hours of the procedure only after:
  - Clear urine is passed
  - She demonstrates no untoward symptoms
  - Stable vital signs have been confirmed

In the IVF laboratory, the harvested ova are classified and graded according to their maturity, on a scale of one to five. The ova are fertilized in a tissue culture medium containing Ham's F-10, supplemented with patient serum, using approximately 50,000 spermatozoa per ovum (in cases of oligospermia, this figure may be doubled or tripled). Recent data have shown that zona drilling and stripping techniques may assist spermatozoa to penetrate the egg under some circumstances. Approximately 70 to 80 percent of the harvested mature oocytes become fertilized.

Embryos showing fragmentation and ova showing no fertilization are discarded. Cleaving embryos are monitored and, at 36 to 48 hours (usually corresponding to four- to eight-cell stage morulas) are transferred to the patient.

For this procedure:

- The patient is prepared in the lithotomy, or knee-chest, position
- Embryos are loaded into a sterile, inert, transfer catheter in a 0.02 to 0.05 mL culture medium
- A guideline catheter is passed through the cervical canal, followed by the embryo transfer catheter
- The embryos are gently dispersed into the upper uterine fundus
- The catheter is checked to confirm that the embryos are no longer present
- The patient is kept at bed rest for one to two hours and is then released
- The patient is given progesterone IM injections (25 mg) daily during the secretory/luteal phase and, in some cases, repeat injections of HCG (2,500 to 5,000 IU) every three to four days
- In late secretory/luteal phase, if pregnancy is suggested by elevated βHCG, levels of βHCG are measured every 48 hours; a rising trend of βHCG confirms pregnancy. If pregnancy is confirmed:
  - The patient is counseled to restrict physical activities

- At approximately five and one-half to six weeks, a pelvic ultrasound (often with a vaginal probe) is performed to confirm the presence of a clinical intrauterine pregnancy

If pregnancy does not occur the couple is supported emotionally, counseled, and advised to:

- Consider repeat IVF after one to two menstrual cycles
- Be aware of treatment independent pregnancy (TIP) which occasionally occurs during non-treatment months

Recent Innovations

There is evidence that super-ovulation via GnRH agonist plus HMG may facilitate the harvesting of many healthy ova in a single stimulation cycle. If multiple ova are obtained and 10 to 15 are fertilized, the transfer of three embryos may be facilitated at the initial attempt and, if embryos are cryopreserved, two further attempts may be completed in later cycles. Australian workers have shown that this innovation may enable a patient to undergo six transfer cycles in a year using ova yielded at only two harvest cycles. The anticipated pregnancy rate is about 40 to 50 percent.

GnRH agonist therapy has played a major role in accomplishing multiple ovulations while avoiding premature LH surges. However, despite initial enthusiasm for this agent, it is not the panacea for all patients. Further data must be gathered to assess the actual place of GnRH agonist therapy in individual patient protocols.

Innovative techniques of zona splitting and zona drilling have been noted to facilitate fertilization by spermatozoa that were otherwise incapable of fertilization.

Recently, many pregnancies have been documented in females whose husbands presented with high levels of antisperm auto-antibodies. Currently, there is hope that these patients may, in the future, be helped with this type of assisted reproductive technology (ART).

As a general rule, IVF is reserved for those in whom prior and simpler methods of conception have failed. It is utilized after failure of supplemented ovulation induction in patients with healthy-appearing oviducts who have been diagnosed as "idiopathic infertile."

Related Techniques

GIFT

See Section #29.

ZIFT/TET

In ZIFT (zygote intrafallopian transfer)/TET (tubal embryo transfer), a variation of the GIFT procedure, IVF is first completed (see above) and the formation of a zygote (or cleaving embryo) is confirmed. The zygote is then transferred into the fallopian tube.

BASIC METHODOLOGY

ZIFT/TET is a two-stage procedure. Prior to the procedure, multiple ovulation induction is stimulated with HMG/HCG. Ova are harvested by transvaginal egg retrieval, ie, vaginal aspiration of the follicles. The ova are then inseminated and fertilized in the laboratory using routine IVF procedures. After fertilization is confirmed, laparoscopy is performed to transfer the early zygotes or embryos into the fallopian tube (12 to 24 hours later for ZIFT and 24 to 48 hours later for TET).

Comment

These methods are advantageous because they provide the opportunity to confirm diagnostic IVF in a particular couple and to ensure that the partner's sperm is capable of fertilizing the patient's ova. Additionally, they provide evidence to a couple that fertilization has taken place, allow couples to take advantage of the patient's healthy fallopian tubes and offer timely transfer of embryos in a most physiological manner.

Preliminary data suggest that, under certain circumstances and in selected patients, higher success rates may be achieved with these methods than with others, particularly in cases of significant semen impairment. However, until such time as ZIFT and TET are confirmed to be significantly more successful than IVF or GIFT in producing live births, these procedures will remain under scrutiny because of their necessary duplication of surgical procedures (though the procedures are minor) and the potential hazard of increased morbidity. The ZIFT and TET techniques appear to be most useful for the couple with a major male fertility problem (oligospermia).

Fiscal/Insurance Considerations

Insurance companies have generally taken a stance to ignore reproductive disorders, by declaring infertility a non-disease entity. This appalling circumstance has resulted in a need for all couples to spend tremendous amounts of their salaries on childbearing attempts. This author believes that disorders of the reproductive system are true medical pathological entities that should be covered by medical insurance in accordance with the coverage afforded all other systems of the body (cardiovascular, respiratory, gastrointestinal, etc.). Non-recognition of reproductive disorders as worthy of insurance coverage has resulted in extreme limitation of the application of costly techniques, such as IVF, to couples desiring children.

In some states, enlightened insurance companies have provided coverage for couples who have no other means of possible conception, affording them the opportunity of two or three IVF attempts. However, an inquiry into 169 IVF centers in 1986-87 indicated that only half of the centers polled were ever successful in producing a viable pregnancy. This was an appalling revelation. It seems clear that IVF centers must be registered and credentialed within the medical community, as is the practice within the American Fertility Society. It is hoped that, once centers are registered, documentation of their capability of affording or achieving pregnancy by IVF can be made and insurance coverage will be forthcoming.

The overall status of ART is changing, literally, from month to month. Indeed, ART now constitutes a total forum and subgroup within the American Fertility Society. Clearly, the advent of these technologies has provided childbearing possibilities for couples who, in the past, were offered absolutely no hope of achieving pregnancy.

However, careful selection and detailed assessment of the feasibility of ART for particular individuals must be continued. Regrettably, some couples do not qualify for IVF due to:

- Absolutely inadequate sperm
- Total obliteration of the uterine cavity
- Non-accessibility of the uterine cavity
- Recurrent chronic infection (eg, tuberculosis)
- Inability to achieve:
    - Adequate ovulatory stimulation
    - Follicular maturation
    - Ovum harvesting

Couples with these infertility problems must be counseled and directed to cease treatment and consider an alternative, such as adoption.

NOTES

APPENDIX – Medications Commonly Used In Infertility

Generic Name	Trade Name	Manufacturer	Common Usage	Suggested Starting Dose
Amoxicillin	Multiple	Multiple	Males: Susceptible organisms at sperm culture	500 mg PO TID or QID X 10 days
Ampicillin	Multiple	Multiple	Females: For antibiotic prophylaxis in pelvic irrigation at surgery (after excluding penicillin sensitivity)	100 mg/L Ringer's lactate solution
Ofloxacin	Floxin	Ortho	Male/Female: Antibiotic treatment of sexually transmitted diseases, ie, gonorrhea, chlamydia	300 mg bid for 7 days
Atropine sulphate	Atropine Sulphate Injection	Elkins-Sinn	Females: As premedication IM 30 minutes before HSG or endometrial biopsy	0.4 mg IM, usually contraindicated in cardiac patients (eg, with mitral valve prolapse)

Benzocaine	Hurricaine (20% Benzocaine)	Beutlich	Females: As topical anesthetic spray to cervix and cervical canal before HSG and endometrial biopsy	Two sprays to cervix and single application to cervical canal
Bromocriptine mesylate	Parlodel	Sandoz	Females: For ovulation induction, patients with hyperprolactinemia or prolactinomas	2.5 mg at bedtime; dose increased weekly until prolactin level is normal
Calcium carbonate	Biocal Calcet Calcium Carbonate	Miles, Inc. Consumer Healthcare Div. Mission Roxane	Females: As supplement for muscle cramps for patients on danazol or GnRH therapy or as estrogen supplementation in hypoestrogenic patients	1 g/day

Generic Name	Trade Name	Manufacturer	Common Usage	Suggested Starting Dose
Calcium citrate	Citracal	Mission	Females: As prophylaxis against calcium loss for patients on GnRH agonists therapy, eg, Lupron®, Synarel®	1,000 mg to 1,500 mg daily
Calcium gluconate	Calcet Calcium gluconate	Mission Roxane		1,000 mg daily
Calcium lactate	Calcet Calphosan	Mission Glenwood		1,000 mg daily
Clomiphene citrate	Clomid Serophene	Marion Merrell Dow Serono	Females: For ovulation induction	50 mg daily X five days beginning on third to fifth day of menstrual cycle (1/2 tab in low body weight [< 105 lbs.] patients)

Danazol	Danocrine	Winthrop	Females: For endometriosis, minimum course three months	400 mg BID or 200 mg QID should lower plasma E_2 below 40 pg/mL by six weeks
Dexamethasone	Decacron Dexamethasone	Merck Sharp & Dohme Roxane	Females: For adrenal hyperandrogenism and/or assisted ovulation induction. Commonly used with clomiphene citrate	0.5 mg at bedtime with snack
Dexamethasone sodium phosphate	Decadon L.A. Dexamethasone Sodium Phosphate Injection Hexadrol	Merck Sharp & Dohme Elkins-Sinn Organon	Females: As perioperative corticosteroid administration, for intraperitoneal lavage, IM injections	20 mg intraperitoneal 20 mg IM, 5 mg to 10 mg IM; Six hourly X four to six doses (dependent on body weight)

Generic Name	Trade Name	Manufacturer	Common Usage	Suggested Starting Dose
Dextran 70	Hyskon	Pharmacia	Females: For intrapertoneal installation at microsurgery During operative hystero-scopy	Less than 150 mL 50 mL to 150 mL High molecular weight sugar (rare allergies, including pulmonary syndromes and DIC)
Doxycycline	Multiple	Multiple	Males/Females: For treatment of chlamydia Females: As perioperative antibiotic prophylaxis	100 mg BID X 21 days 200 mg IV diluted in 250 mL and buffered to reduce incidence of phlebitis
Erythromycin	ERYC E-Mycin Ery-Tabs Erythromycin Ethylsuccinate	Parke-Davis Boots Abbott Lederle	Males/Females: For chlamydial infections not responsive to doxycyclines Females: As intraoperative irrigation solutions in	250 mg to 400 mg TID X 14 days 100 mg/L heparinized Ringer's lactate solution

			patients allergic to penicillin	
Estradiol	Estrace	Mead Johnson	Females: As supplement to clomiphene citrate when antiestrogen effects cause reduction in or absence of cervical mucus	1 mg to 2 mg daily on days eight through 14 of cycle
Estrogens, conjugated	Premarin	Wyeth-Ayerst		0.625 mg to 1.25 mg daily X seven days
Ethinyl estradiol	Estinyl	Schering		.02 mg to .06 mg daily on days eight through 14 of cycle (of ovulation induction)
Glucagon	Glucogon	Lilly	Females: For non-atropinized patients with apparent cornual spasm at HSG; action at one minute, lasting ± 10 to 30 minutes	0.5 mg/mL to 1 mg/mL diluted and slow IV injection (beef, pork pancreatic extract-protein; rare allergies)

Generic Name	Trade Name	Manufacturer	Common Usage	Suggested Starting Dose
GnRH (Synthetic LH-RH):				
Gonadorelin hydrochloride	Factrel	Ayerst	Male/Female: Diagnostic single injection evaluation of pituitary-gonadotropin response	100 mcg IV or subcutaneous
Gonadorelin acetate	Lutrepulse	Ortho	Male/Female: Pulsatile intravenous injection via the pump system for induction of ovulation in patients with primary hypothalamic amenorrhea and selected cases of polycystic ovarian disease	5 mcg per 90 to 120/sec. interval pulsatile therapy via computerized pump; close observation is still advisable
GnRH Agonists:				
Leuprolide acetate	Lupron	TAP	Females: For controlled ovarian stimulation and avoidance of premature LH	0.5 mg to 1 mg daily from ± day 24 of previous cycle on contraception;

			surge, for endometriosis inadequately suppressed by danazol, and as preoperative suppression for fibroid surgery	commenced on day one in some circumstances; 1 mg daily two to six months Prophylactic calcium supplements 1000 mg/day, 1 mg daily two to six months (calcium supplements as above)
GnRH Agonists: Nafarelin acetate	Synarel	Syntex	Females: Approved for use in endometriosis. Also used for uterine fibroids and preparation for ovulation induction—IVF, GIFT, ZIFT	400 μg daily as 200 μg BID; intranasal spray

Generic Name	Trade Name	Manufacturer	Common Usage	Suggested Starting Dose
Gonadotropins (Human Menopausal [HMG])	Pergonal	Serono	Females: For ovulation induction, supplemented ovulation induction, and monitoring of ovarian hyperstimulation (ART, GIFT or IVF)	Individualized regimens dependent on clinical and endocrine circumstances
Gonadotropin (Human Chorionic [HCG])	Pregnyl Profasi	Organon Serono	Females: To replace or supplement LH surge to "trigger" ovulation	5,000 to 10,000 IU IM in 1 mL to 2 mL diluent Close monitoring, usually with cervical exam, E_2 and ultrasound. Contraindicated and withheld if hyperstimulation syndrome anticipated

Guaifenesin	Humibid L.A. Scot-Tussin Expectorant	Adams Scot-Tussin	Females: To increase cervical mucus for patients on clomiphene citrate with inadequate mucus response	600 mg tabs one to two BID X five days, days nine through 13 100 mg (1 tsp) TID days nine to 13 of cycle
Methyl-testosterone	Metandren Linguets	CIBA	Males: For asthenospermia in selected cases	5 mg to 10 mg sublingual daily X 30 to 60 days
Norgestrel	Lo/Ovral Ovral	Wyeth-Ayerst	Females: As suppressive therapy for functional ovarian cysts and endometriosis, if fiscal constraints for danazol or GnRH agonist therapy exist	One daily for 25 to 40 days

Generic Name	Trade Name	Manufacturer	Common Usage	Suggested Starting Dose
Povidone iodine	Betadine Skin Cleanser	Purdue Frederick	Females: As standard cervical, vaginal, perineal and abdominal preparation for all minor and major surgeries (after excluding iodine allergy)	Standard dose
Prednisone	Deltasone Prednisone	Upjohn Multiple	Females: For adrenal hyperandrogenism	5 mg at bedtime with snack days two to 16 or throughout menstrual cycle
Progesterone	Progesterone 50	Legere	Females: For luteal phase deficiency presenting as ovulatory dysfunction or recurrent early pregnancy loss, for proven deficiency for patients on blood progesterones, and at en-	25 mg BID two days after temperature rise for 12 days, suppository form

			dometrial biopsy for patients with repeated late luteal phase defect	
Progestins:				
Medroxyprogesterone acetate	Provera tablets Amen tabs Curretab	Upjohn Carnrick Reid-Rowell	Females: For progestogen withdrawal bleeding in patients with anovulatory "estrus" state	10 mg daily for five days; contraindicated in pregnancy
	Cycrin	Wyeth-Ayerst	Females: Progestogen supplementation in patients on estrogen replacement therapy; progestin suppression for endometriosis	10 mg daily for 13 days (days 13 to 25 of cycle)
Megestrol acetate	Megace	Bristol-Meyers	Females: For progestin suppression for patients with endometriosis	20 mg to 40 mg BID for 90 to 120 days

Generic Name	Trade Name	Manufacturer	Common Usage	Suggested Starting Dose
Norethindrone acetate	Aygestin Norlutate	Wyeth-Ayerst Parke-Davis	Females: For progestogen supplementation for patients on estrogen replacement therapy	5 mg daily for 13 days
Tetracycline hydrochloride	Multiple	Multiple	Females: As common antibiotic prophylaxis at HSG	500 mg PO QID one day before and three days after procedure. All patients should be proven chlamydial culture negative before HSG
Thyroid thyroxine	Synthroid	Boots-Flint	Males/Females: As thyroid replacement therapy for patients with hypothyroidism	.05 daily; dosage adjusted by 0.025 every two to three weeks; monitored by clinical response and TSH, T_3 and T_4

Urofollitropin (FSH)	Metrodin	Serono (75 IU/mL)	Females: As purified extract of FSH for ovulation induction, classically for multiple ovulation induction for GIFT and/or IVF	1 to 2 ampules/day on days two through four of cycle, in combination with HMG therapy
Vasopressin	Pitressin	Parke-Davis	Females: In selected cases of microsurgery, cornual dissection, anastomosis, unruptured ectopic pregnancy, and fibroids (at myomectomy)	Five units diluted in 30 mL saline, topical injection 1 mL to 5 mL Minimal dose necessary to achieve hemostatic effect; close cardiovascular monitoring essential

References

Abraham GE: Ovarian and adrenal contribution to peripheral androgens during menstrual cycle. J Clin Endocrinol Metab 1974;389:340.

Alexander NJ, Anderson DJ: Immunology of semen. In: Modern Trends in Infertility and Conception Control. Wallach EE, Kempers RD (eds.) Chicago: Year Book Medical Publishers, 1988;4:445-458.

Alexander NM, Anderson DJ: Vasectomy: Consequences of autoimmunity to sperm antigens. Fertil Steril 1979;32:253.

Amelar RD: Coagulation, liquefaction and viscosity of human semen. J Urol 1962;87:187.

Amelar RD, Hotchkiss RS: The split ejaculate. Fertil Steril 1965;16:46.

Andrews WC, et al: The American Fertility Society revised classification of endometriosis. Fertil Steril 1985;43:3.

Asch R, Balmaceda J, Rochester M: Pregnancy following GIFT (gamete intrafallopian transfer) in premature ovarian failure. Presented at the Conjoint Annual Meeting of The American Fertility Society, the Canadian Fertility and Andrology Fertility Society, Toronto, Canada, September 27 to October 2, 1986. Published by The American Fertility Society, in the abstracts of the scientific paper and poster sessions, 1986;54.

Ayers JWT: Differential response to adrenocorticotropin hormone stimulation in polycystic ovarian disease with high and low dehydroepiandrosterone sulfate levels. Fertil Steril 1982;37:645.

Barbieri RL, Evans S, Kistner RW: Danazol in the treatment of endometriosis: Analysis of 100 cases with a 4-year follow-up. Fertil Steril 1982;37:737.

Bardin CW, Lipset M: Testosterone and androstenedione blood production rates in normal women and women with idiopathic hirsutism and polycystic ovaries. J Clin Invest 1967;46:891.

Barwin BN: Intrauterine insemination of husband's semen. J Reprod Fertil 1978;36:101.

Behrman SJ, Kistner RW, Patton GW, Jr (eds.): Progress In Infertility. Boston/Toronto: Little, Brown & Co., Inc., 1988.

Blackwell RE: Diagnosis and management of prolactinomas. In: Modern Trends In Infertility and Conception Control. Wallach EE, Kempers Rd (eds.) Chicago: Year Book Medical Publishers, 1988;4:197-208.

Blasco L: Clinical tests of sperm fertilizing ability. Fertil Steril 1984;41:177.

Brodie BL, Wentz AC: Late onset congenital adrenal hyperplasia: A gynecologist's perspective. In: Modern Trends In Infertility and Conception Control. Wallach EE, Kempers RD (eds.) Chicago: Year Book Medical Publishers, 1988;4:135-146.

Bronson R, Cooper G, Rosenfield D: Sperm antibodies: Their role in infertility. Fertil Steril 1984;42:171.

Brosens IA, Koninckx PR, Corvelyn PA: A study of plasma progesterone, oestradiol-17β, prolactin and LH levels, and the luteal phase appearance of the ovaries in patients with endometriosis and infertility. Br J Obstet Gynecol 1978;85:246.

Bruhat MA, Kase N: Treatment of ectopic pregnancy by means of laparoscopy. Fertil Steril 1980;33:411.

Bukovsky I, Langer R, et al: Conservative surgery for tubal pregnancy. Obstet Gynecol 1979;53:709.

Buster JE, Bustillo M, et al: Nonsurgical transfer of in vitro fertilization donated ova to five infertile women: Report of two pregnancies. Lancet 1983;2:223.

Butler L, Wilson E, et al: Collaborative study of pregnancy rates following danazol therapy of stage I endometriosis. Fertil Steril 1984;41:373.

Buttram VC Jr: Conservative surgery for endometriosis in the infertile female: A study of 206 patients with implications for both medical and surgical therapy. Fertil Steril 1982;31:117.

Buttram VC, et al: The American Fertility Society classification of adnexal adhesions. Fertil Steril 1988;49:6.

Buttram VC Jr, Reiter RC, Ward S: Treatment of endometriosis with danazol: Report of a 6-year prospective study. Fertil Steril 1985;43:353.

Chang MC: Fertilizing capacity of spermatozoa deposited into the fallopian tubes. Nature 1951;168:697.

Chang MC: The meaning of sperm capacitation: A historical perspective. J Androl 1984;5:45.

Charny CW: Clomiphene therapy in male infertility: A negative report. Fertil Steril 1979;32:551.

Chong AP, Taymor ML: Sixteen years' experience with therapeutic donor insemination. Fertil Steril 1975;26:791.

Clinical Gynecologic Endocrinology and Infertility: Speroff L, Glass RH, Kase NG (eds.) Baltimore: Williams and Wilkins Co., 1978.

Cohen BM: Microsurgical reconstruction of congenital tubal anomalies. Microsurg 1987;8:68-77.

Cohen BM: Surgery of the ovary including anatomic derangements of the fimbrial-gonadal ovum-capture mechanism. In: Atlas of Female Infertility Surgery. Hunt RB (ed.) Chicago: Year Book Medical Publishers, Inc., 1986.

Cohen BM: Surgical management of infertility in the polycystic ovary syndrome. In: The Infertile Female. Givens JR, et al (eds.) Chicago: Year Book Medical Publishers, Inc., 1979.

Cohen BM, Katz M: The significance of the convoluted oviduct in the infertile woman. J Reprod Med 1978;21:31.

Cohen J, Simons RF, et al: Factors affecting survival and implantation of cryopreserved human embryos. J Vitro Embryo Trans 1986;3:46.

Cohen J, Simons RF, et al: In vitro fertilization: A treatment for male infertility. Fertil Steril 1985;43:422.

Cohen J, Simons RF, et al: Pregnancies following the frozen storage of expanding human blastocysts. J Vitro Fertil Embryo Trans 1985;2:59.

Cohen J, Weber RFA, et al: In vitro fertilizing capacity of human spermatozoa with the use of zone-free hamster ova: Interassay variation and prognostic value. Fertil Steril 1982;37:565.

Cohen MR: Intrauterine insemination. Int J Fertil 1962;7:235.

Crowley WF, Comite F, et al: Therapeutic use of pituitary desensitization with a long-acting LHRH agonist: A potential new treatment for idiopathic precocious puberty. J Clin Endocrinol Metab 1981;52:370.

Csapo AI, Pulkkinen MO, Wiest WO: Effects of luteectomy and progesterone replacement therapy in early pregnant patients. Am J Obstet Gynecol 1973;115:759.

Damewood MD, Grochow LB: Prospects for fertility after chemotherapy or radiation for neoplastic disease. In: Modern Trends in Infertility and Conception Control. Wallach EE, Kempers RD (eds.) Chicago: Year Book Medical Publishers, 1988;4:63-79.

Daniell JF: The role of lasers in infertility surgery. In: Modern Trends in Infertility and Conception Control. Wallach EE, Kempers RD (eds.) Chicago: Year Book Medical Publishers, 1988;4:295-303.

Daniell JF: The role of lasers in infertility surgery. Fertil Steril 1984;42:815.

Daniell JF, Christianson C: Combined laparoscopic surgery and danazol therapy for pelvic endometriosis. Fertil Steril 1981;35:521.

Davajan V, Vargyas JM, et al: Abstract: Intrauterine insemination with washed sperm to treat infertility. Fertil Steril 1983;40:419.

Dawood MY, Raghavan KS: Oxytocin during human pregnancy and parturition. Obstet Gynecol 1978;51:138.

DeCherney AH, Boyes SP: Isthmic ectopic pregnancy segmental resection as the treatment of choice. Fertil Steril 1985;44:30.

DeCherney AH, Kase N: The conservative surgical management of unruptured ectopic pregnancy. Obstet Gynecol 1979;54:451.

DeCherney AH, Kort H, et al: Increased pregnancy rate with oil soluble hysterosalpingography dye. Fertil Steril 1980;33:407.

DeCherney AH, Romero R, Naftolin F: Surgical management of unruptured ectopic pregnancy. Fertil Steril 1981;35:2.

Diamond E: Lysis of postoperative pelvic adhesions in infertility. Fertil Steril 1979;31:287.

Diamond MP, Christianson C, et al: Pregnancy following use of the cervical cap for home artificial insemination utilizing homologous semen. Fertil Steril 1983;39:480.

di Zerega GS, Marut EL, et al: Asymmetrical ovarian function during recruitment and selection of the dominant follicle in the menstrual cycle of the rhesus monkey. J Clin Endocrinol Metab 1980;51:698.

Dmowski WP, Cohen MR: Antigonadotropin (danazol) in the treatment of endometriosis: Evaluation of post-treatment fertility and three-year follow-up data. Am J Obstet Gynecol 1978;130:41.

Dmowski WP, Cohen MR: Treatment of endometriosis with an antigonadotropin, danazol: A laparoscopic and histologic evaluation. Obstet Gynecol 1975;45:147.

Dmowski WP, Gaynor L, et al: Artificial insemination homologous with oligospermic semen separated on albumin columns. Fertil Steril 1979;31:58.

Drake TS, Tredqay DR: Spontaneous pregnancy during the infertility evaluation. Fertil Steril 178;30:36.

Dubin L, Amelar RA: Varicocelectomy as therapy in male infertility: A study of 504 cases. Fertil Steril 1975;26:217.

Edwards RG, Steptoe PC, Purdy JM: Fertilization and cleavage in vitro of preovulatory human oocytes. Nature 1970;227:1307.

Engel T, Jewelewicz R, et al: Ovarian hyperstimulation syndrome: Report of a case with notes on pathogenesis and treatment. Am J Obstet Gynecol 1972;112:1052.

The Ethics Committee of The American Fertility Society: Ethical considerations of the new reproductive technologies. Fertil Steril (Suppl 1) 1986;46:1S.

Fayez JA: An assessment of the role of operative laparoscopy in tuboplasty. Fertil Steril 1983;39:476.

Frisch RE, McArthur JW: Menstrual cycles: Fatness as a determinant of minimum weight for height necessary for their maintenance or onset. Science 1974;185:949.

Garcia JE, Acosta AA, et al: Advanced endometrial maturation after ovulation induction with human menopausal gonadotropin/human chorionic gonadotropin for in vitro fertilization. Fertil Steril 1984;41:31.

Garcia JE, Jones GS, et al: Human menopausal gonadotropin/ human chorionic gonadotropin follicular maturation for oocyte aspiration: Phase I, 1981. Fertil Steril 1983;39:167.

Garcia JE, Jones GS, et al: Human menopausal gonadotropin/ human chorionic gonadotropin follicular maturation for oocyte aspiration: Phase II, 1981. Fertil Steril 1983;39:174.

Gindoff PR, Jewelewicz R: Reproductive potential in the older woman. In: Modern Trends in Infertility and Conception Control. Wallach EE, Kempers RD (eds.) Chicago: Year Book Medical Publishers, 1988;4:7-19.

Givens JR, Andersen RN, et al: The effectiveness of two oral contraceptives in suppressing plasma androstenedione, testosterone, LH and FSH, and in stimulating plasma testosterone-binding capacity in hirsute women. Am J Obstet Gynecol 1976;124:333.

Glass RH, Ericksson RJ: Intrauterine insemination of isolated motile sperm. Fertil Steril 1978;29:535.

Glass RH, Golbus MS: Habitual abortion. Fertil Steril 1978;29:257.

Goldstein D, Zuckerman H, et al: Correlation between estradiol and progesterone in cycles with luteal phase deficiency. Fertil Steril 1982;37:348.

Gomel V: Laparoscopic tubal surgery in infertility. Obstet Gynecol 1975;47:47.

Gomel V: Microsurgery in female infertility. Boston: Little, Brown & Co., 1983;80.

Gomel V: Microsurgical reversal of female sterilization: A reappraisal. Fertil Steril 1980;33:587.

Gomel V: Salpingo-ovariolysis by laparoscopy in infertility. Fertil Steril 1983;40:607.

Gomel V: Salpingostomy by laparoscopy in the infertile patient. J Reprod Med 1977;18:265.

Gomel V: Tubal reanastomosis by microsurgery. Fertil Steril 1977;28:59.

Gomel V, Swolin K: Salpingostomy: Microsurgical technique and results. Clin Obstet Gynecol 1980;23:1203.

Greenglatt RM, Handsfield HH, et al: Screening therapeutic insemination donors for sexually transmitted diseases: Overview and recommendations. Fertil Steril 1986;46:351.

Guzick DS, Rock JA: A comparison of danazol and conservative surgery for the treatment of infertility due to mild or moderate endometriosis. Fertil Steril 1983;40:580.

Haas GG Jr, Beer AE: Immunologic influences on reproductive biology: Sperm gametogenesis and maturation in the male and female genital tracts. In: Modern Trends in Infertility and Conception Control. Wallach EE, Kempers RD (eds.) Chicago: Year Book Medical Publishers, 1988;4:459-471.

Hafez ESE, Evans TN (eds.): Human Reproduction Conception and Contraception. New York: Harper & Row Publishers, Inc., 1973.

Halbert SA, Tam PY, Blandau RJ: Egg transport in the rabbit oviduct: The roles of cilia and muscle. Science 1976;191:1052.

Haney AF, Misukonis MA, Weinberg JB: Macrophages and infertility: Oviductal macrophages as potential mediators of infertility. Fertil Steril 1983;39:310.

Hardy J, Beauregard H, Robert F: Prolactin-secreting pituitary adenomas: Transsphenoidal microsurgical treatment. In: Progress in Prolactin Physiology and Pathology. Robyn C, Harter M (eds.) Elsevier-North Holland, Amsterdam, 1978;361-369.

Hargrove JT, Abraham GE: Abnormal luteal function in endometriosis. Fertil Steril 1980;34:302.

Hasson HM: Electrocoagulation of pelvic endometriotic lesions of endometriosis at laparoscopy for infertility. Am J Obstet Gynecol 1979;135:115.

Hodgen GD: Surrogate embryo transfer combined with estrogen-progesterone therapy in monkeys, implantation, gestation and delivery without ovaries. JAMA 1983;250:2167.

Hopkins CC, Hall JE, Santoro NF, et al: Closed intravenous administration of gonadotropin-releasing hormone: safety of extended peripheral intravenous catheterization. Obstet Gynecol 1989;74:267-270.

Horne HW, Clyman M, et al: The prevention of postoperative pelvic adhesions following conservative operative treatment for human infertility. Internat J Fertil 1983;18:109.

Hulka JF: Adnexal adhesions: A prognostic staging and classification system based on a five-year survey of fertility surgery results at Chapel Hill. Am J Obstet Gynecol 1982;144:141.

Insler V, Melmed H, et al: The cervical score. Int J Gynaecol Obstet 1972;10:223.

Isojima S, Li T, Ashitaka Y: Immunologic analysis of sperm immobilizing factor found in serum of women with unexplained infertility. Am J Obstet Gynecol 1968;101:677.

Jacobs HS, Knuth UA, et al: Postpill amenorrhea, cause or coincidence? Br Med J 1977;2:940.

Jones HW Jr, Acosta AA, et al: Three years of in vitro fertilization at Norfolk. Fertil Steril 1984;42:826.

Jones HW Jr, Rock JA: On the reanastomosis of the fallopian tubes after surgical sterilization. Fertil Steril 1978;29:702.

Judd HL, Yen SCC: Serum androstenedione and testosterone levels during the menstrual cycle. J Clin Endocrinol Metab 1973;38:475.

Judd HL, Rigg LA, et al: The effects of ovarian wedge resection on circulating gonadotropin and ovarian steroid levels in patients with polycystic ovary syndrome. J Clin Endocrinol Metab 1976;3:347.

Katz M, Carr PJ, et al: Hormonal effects on wedge resection of polycystic ovaries. Obstet Gynecol 1978;51:437.

Kerin JFP, Peek J, et al: Improved conception rate after intrauterine insemination of washed spermatozoa from men with poor quality semen. Lancet 1984;1:553.

Keye WR, Watson GA, Dixon J: The use of the argon laser in the treatment of experimental endometriosis. Fertil Steril 1983;39:26.

Kistner RW: Management of endometriosis in the infertile patient. Fertil Steril 1975;26:1151.

Kleinberg DL, Noel GL, Frantz AG: Galactorrhea: A study of 235 cases, including 48 with pituitary tumors. N Engl J Med 1977;296:589.

Knobil E: The neuroendocrine control of the menstrual cycle. Recent Prog Horm Res 1980;36:53.

Kremer J: A new technique for intrauterine insemination. Int J Fertil 1979;24:53.

Lavy G, Diamond MP, DeCherney AH: Ectopic pregnancy: Its relationship to tubal reconstructive surgery. In: Modern Trends in Infertility and Conception Control. Wallach EE, Kempers RD (eds.) Chicago: Year Book Medical Publishers, 1988;4:281-294.

Levine RL: Economic impact of pelviscopic surgery. J Reprod Med 1985;30:655.

Lipshultz LI: Beyond the routine semen analysis. Fertil Steril 1982;38:153.

Lipshultz LI, Cunningham GR, Howards SS: Differential diagnosis in male infertility. In: Infertility in the Male. Lipshultz LI, Howards SS (eds.) New York: Churchill Livingstone, 1983;249.

Lipshultz LI, Howards SS: Evaluation of the subfertile male. In: Infertility in the Male. Lipshultz LI, Howards SS (eds.) New York: Churchill Livingstone, 1983;187.

Lobo RA, Paul WL, Goebelsmann U: Dehydroepiandrosterone sulfate as an indicator of adrenal androgen function. Obstet Gynecol 1981;57:69.

Mackey RA, Glass RH, et al: Pregnancy following hysterosalpingography with oil and water soluble dye. Fertil Steril 1971;22:504.

MacLeod J: Human male infertility. Obstet Gynecol Surv 1971;26:335.

MacLeod J: Human seminal cytology as a sensitive indicator of the germinal epithelium. Int J Fertil 1964;9:281.

MacLeod J, Gold RZ: The male factor in fertility and infertility: Spermatozoan counts in 1000 cases of known fertility and in 1000 cases of infertile marriages. J Urol 1951;66:436.

Mahesh VB, Bratlid D, Lindabeck T: Hormone levels following wedge resection in polycystic ovary syndrome. Obstet Gynecol 1978;51:64.

Mahlstedt PP: The psychological component of infertility. In: Modern Trends in Infertility and Conception Control. Wallach EE, Kempers RD (eds.) Chicago: Year Book Medical Publishers, 1988;4:107-118.

Malinak LR: Infertility and endometriosis: Operative technique, clinical staging, and prognosis. Clin Obstet Gynecol 1980;23:925.

March CM, Goebelsmann U, et al: Roles of estradiol and progesterone in eliciting the mid-cycle luteinizing hormone and follicle-stimulating hormone surges. J Clin Endocrinol Metab 1979;49:507.

March CM, Israel R, March AD: Hysteroscopic management of intrauterine adhesions. Am J Obstet Gynecol 1978;130:653.

Martin DC: CO2 laser laparoscopy for treatment of endometriosis associated with infertility. J Reprod Med 1985;3:409.

Marut EL, Williams RF, et al: Pulsatile pituitary gonadotropin secretion during maturation of the dominant follicle in monkeys: Estrogen positive feedback enhances the biological activity of LH. Endocrin 1981;109:2270.

McComb P, Gomel V: Cornual occlusion and its microsurgical reconstruction. Clin Obstet Gynecol 1980;23:1229.

McNatty KP, Baird YS, et al: Androgen biosynthesis in human ovarian follicles; cellular source, gonadotropic control, and adenosine -3', 5'-cyclic monophosphate mediation. J Clin Endocrinol Metab 1978;76:527.

McNatty KP, Makris A, et al: The production of progesterone, androgens, and estrogens by granulosa cells, thecal tissue, and stromal tissue from human ovaries in vitro. J Clin Endocrinol Metab 1979;49:687.

McNatty KP, Smith DM, et al: The intraovarian sites of androgen and estrogen formation in women with normal and hyperandrogenic ovaries as judged by in vitro experiments. J Clin Endocrinol Metab 1980;50:755.

McNatty KP, Smith DM, et al: The microenvironment of the human antral follicle: Interrelationships among the steroid levels in antral fluid, the population of granulosa cells, and the status of the oocyte in vivo and in vitro. J Clin Endocrinol Metab 1951;49:851.

Meldrum DR, Abraham GE: Peripheral and ovarian venous concentrations of various steroid hormones in virilizing ovarian tumors. Obstet Gynecol 1979;53:36.

Meldrum DR, Chang RJ, et al: "Medical Oophorectomy" using a long-acting GnRH agonist: A possible new approach to the treatment of endometriosis. J Clin Endocrinol Metab 1982;54:1081.

Menge AC, Medley NE, et al: The incidence and influence of antisperm antibodies in infertile human couples on sperm-cervical mucus interactions and subsequent fertility. Fertil Steril 1982;38:439.

Menon V, Butt WR, Clayton RN, et al: Pulsatile administration of GnRH for the treatment of hypogonadotropic hypogonadism. Clin Endocrinol 1984;21:223-232.

Moghissi KS, Boyce CR: Management of endometriosis with oral medroxyprogesterone acetate. Obstet Gynecol 1976; 47:265.

Moghissi KS, Syner FN, Evans TN: A composite picture of the menstrual cycle. Am J Obstet Gynecol 1972;114:405.

Muasher SJ, Garcia JE, Rosenwaks Z: The combination of follicle-stimulating hormone and human menopausal gonadotropin for the induction of multiple follicular maturation for in vitro fertilization. Fertil Steril 1985;44:62.

Murphy AA: Operative laparoscopy. In: Modern Trends In Infertility and Conception Control. Wallach EE, Kempers RD (eds.) Chicago: Year Book Medical Publishers, 1988;4:263-280.

Muse KN, Wilson EA: How does mild endometriosis cause infertility? Fertil Steril 1982;38:145.

Navot D, Laufer N, et al: Artificially-induced endometrial cycles and establishment of pregnancies in the absence of ovaries. N Engl J Med 1986;314:806.

Novak ER, Jones GS, Jones HW: Novak's Textbook of Gynecology, 9th edition. Baltimore: The Williams and Wilkins Co., 1976.

Noyes RW, Hertig AT, Rock J: Dating the endometrial biopsy. Fertil Steril 1950;1:3.

Overstreet JW, Yanagimachi R, et al: Penetration of human spermatozoa into the human zona pellucida and the zona-free hamster egg: A study of fertile donors and infertile patients. Fertil Steril 1980;33:534.

Patton GW: Pregnancy outcome following microsurgical fimbrioplasty. Fertil Steril 1982;37:150.

Paulson DF: Clomiphene citrate in the management of male hypofertility: Predictors for treatment selection. Fertil Steril 1977;28:1226.

Paulson DF, Wacksman J, et al: Hyperfertility and clomiphene citrate therapy. Fertil Steril 1975;226:982.

Peterson EP, Musich JR, Behrman SJ: Uterotubal implantation and obstetric outcome after previous sterilization. Am J Obstet Gynecol 1977;128:662.

Pittaway DE, Mason W, et al: Luteal phase defects in infertility patients with endometriosis. Fertil Steril 1983;39:712.

Rebar RW, Erikson GF, Yen SSC: Idiopathic premature ovarian failure: Clinical and endocrine characteristics. Fertil Steril 1982;37:35.

Reich H, McGlynn F: Treatment of ovarian endometriomas using laparoscopic surgical techniques. J Reprod Med 1986;31:577.

Ritchie WGM: Ultrasound in the evaluation of normal and induced ovulation. In: Modern Trends in Infertility and Conception Control. Wallach EE, Kempers RD (eds.) Chicago: Year Book Medical Publishers, 1988;4:167-181.

Robert JF, Quigley ME, Yen SSC: Endogenous opiates modulate pulsatile luteinizing hormone release in humans. J Clin Endocrinol Metab 1981;52:583.

Rock JA, Bergquist CA, et al: Tubal anastomosis following unipolar cautery. Fertil Steril 1982;37:613.

Rodriguez-Rigau LJ, Smith DK, Steinberger E: Relationship of varicocele to sperm output and fertility of male partners in infertile couples. Urology 1978;120:691.

Rogers BJ: Hamster egg evaluation of human sperm using in vitro fertilization. In: In Vitro Fertilization and Embryo Transfer. Crosignani PG, Rubin BL (eds.) London, UK: Academic Press, 1983;101.

Rogers JB: The sperm penetration assay: Its usefulness reevaluated. In: Modern Trends in Infertility and Conception Control. Wallach EE, Kempers RD (eds.) Chicago: Year Book Medical Publishers, 1988;4:425-444.

Rosenwaks Z: Donor eggs. In: In Vitro Fertilization, Norfolk. Jones HW Jr, Jones GS, et al (eds.) Baltimore: The Williams and Wilkins Co., 1986;270.

Rosenwaks Z, Veeck LL, Liu HC: Pregnancy following transfer of in vitro fertilized donated oocytes. Fertil Steril 1986;45:417.

Sampson JA: Peritoneal endometriosis due to the menstrual dissemination of endometrial tissue into the peritoneal cavity. Am J Obstet Gynecol 1972;14:422.

Santen RJ, Ruby EB: Enhanced frequency and magnitude of episodic LH-releasing hormone discharge as a hypothalamic mechanism for increased LH secretion. J Clin Endocrinol Metab 1979;48:315.

Saunders DM, Hunter JC, et al: Treatment of luteal phase inadequacy with bromocriptine. Obstet Gynecol 1978;53:287.

Schenken RS, Malinak LR: Conservative surgery versus expectant management for the infertile patient with mild endometriosis. Fertil Steril 1982;37:183.

Schenker JG, Yarkoni S, Granat M: Multiple pregnancies following induction of ovulation. Fertil Steril 1981;35:105.

Schifrin BS, Erez S, Moore JG: Teenage endometriosis. Am J Obstet Gynecol 1973;116:973.

Schlaff WD: Dynamic testing in reproductive endocrinology. In: Modern Trends in Infertility and Conception Control. Wallach EE, Kempers RD (eds.) Chicago: Year Book Medical Publishers, 1988;4:149-166.

Schmidt CL: Endometriosis: A reappraisal of pathogenesis and treatment. In: Modern Trends in Infertility and Conception Control. Wallach EE, Kempers RD (eds.) Chicago: Year Book Medical Publishers, 1988;4:325-341.

Schriock DE, Jaffe RB: Induction of ovulation with gonadotropin-releasing hormone. Obstet Gynecol Sur 1986;41: 414-423.

Schwartz M, Jewelewicz R: The use of gonadotropins for induction of ovulation. Fertil Steril 1981;35:3.

Scialli AR: The reproductive toxicity of ovulation induction. In: Modern Trends In Infertility and Conception Control. Wallach EE, Kempers RD (eds.) Chicago: Year Book Medical Publishers, 1988;4:81-89.

Seibel MM, Berger MJ, et al: The effectiveness of danazol on subsequent fertility in minimal endometriosis. Fertil Steril 1982;38:534.

Seibel MM, McArdle CR, et al: The role of ultrasound in ovulation induction: A critical appraisal. Fertil Steril 1981; 36:573.

Semm K, Mettler L: Technical progress in pelvic surgery via operative laparoscopy. Am J Obstet Gynecol 1980;138:121.

Shangold MM, Gatz ML, Thysen B: Acute effects of exercise on plasma concentrations of prolactin and testosterone in recreational women runners. Fertil Steril 1981;35:699.

Shapiro AG, Thomas T, Epstein M: Management of hyperstimulation syndrome. Fertil Steril 1977;28:237.

Sher G, Knutzen VK, et al: In vitro sperm capacitation and transcervical intrauterine insemination for the treatment of refractory infertility: Phase 1. Fertil Steril 1984;41:260.

Sherins RJ, Howards SS: Male infertility. In: Campbell's Urology, Vol. 1. Walsh PC, Gittles RF, et al (eds.) Philadelphia: WB Saunders, 1986;640.

Shulman S, Harlin B, et al: Immune infertility and new approaches to treatment. Fertil Steril 1978;29:309.

Siegler AM: Hysterosalpingography. New York: Medcon Press, 1974.

Siegler AM, Kontopoulos V: The analysis of macrosurgical and microsurgical techniques in the management of the tuboperitoneal factor in infertility. Fertil Steril 1979;32:377.

Silber SJ, Cohen R: Microsurgical reversal of female sterilization: The role of tubal length. Fertil Steril 1980;33:598.

Soules MR, Moore DE, et al: The relationship between the postcoital test and the sperm penetration assay. Fertil Steril 1982;38:384.

Speroff L, Levin RM, et al: A practical approach for the evaluation of women with abnormal polytomography or elevated prolactin levels. Am J Obstet Gynecol 1979;135:896.

Stein IF: Wedge resection of the ovaries: The Stein-Leventhal syndrome. In: Ovulation. Greenblatt RD (ed.) Philadelphia, PA: J.B. Lippincott Co., 1966;150.

Stein IF, Leventhal ML: Amenorrhea associated with bilateral polycystic ovaries. Am J Obstet Gynecol 1935;29:181.

Stenchever MA, Spandoni LR, et al: Benefits of the sperm (hamster ova) penetration assay in the evaluation of the infertile couple. Am J Obstet Gynecol 1982;143:91.

Steptoe P, Edwards R: Reimplantation of a human embryo with subsequent tubal pregnancy. Lancet 1976;1:880.

Swolin K: Electromicrosurgery and salpingostomy long-term results. Am J Obstet Gynecol 1974;121:418.

Timor-Tritsch IE, Rottem S (eds.): Transvaginal Sonography. New York: Elsevier Science Publishing Co., Inc., 1988.

Trounson A, Freeman L: The use of embryo cryopreservation in human IVF programmes. Clin Obstet Gynecol 1985;12:825.

Trounson A, Leeton J, et al: The investigation of idiopathic infertility by in vitro fertilization. Fertil Steril 1980;34:431.

Trounson A, Leeton J, et al: Pregnancy established in an infertile patient after transfer of a donated embryo fertilized in vitro. Br Med J 1983;286:835.

Trounson A, Leeton J, et al: Successful human pregnancies by in vitro fertilization and embryo transfer in the controlled ovulatory cycle. Science 1981;212:681.

Trounson A, Mohr L: Human pregnancy following cryopreservation, thawing and transfer of an eight-cell embryo. Nature 1983;305:707.

U.S. Department of Health, Education and Welfare (HEW) Ethics Advisory Board: HEW support of research involving human in vitro fertilization and embryo transfer. Federal Regulation 44, 1979;35:033.

Wallach EE, Manara LR, Eisenberg E: Experience with 143 cases of tubal surgery. Fertil Steril 1983;39:609.

Wheeler JM, Malinak LR: Recurrent endometriosis: Incidence, management, and prognosis. Am J Obstet Gynecol 1983;146: 247.

Wild RA, Umstot ES, et al: Adrenal function in hirsutism II: Effect of an oral contraceptive. J Clin Endocrinol Metab 1982;54:676.

Williams RF, Hodgen GD: Disparate effects of human chorionic gonadotropin during the late follicular phase in monkeys: Normal ovulation, follicular atresia, ovarian acyclicity and hypersecretion of follicle-stimulating hormone. Fertil Steril 1980;33:64.

Williams WL: Biochemistry of capacitation of spermatozoa. In: Biology of Mammalian Fertilization and Implantation. Moghissi KS, Hafez ESE (eds.) Springfield: IL: Charles C. Thomas, 1972.

Winston RLM: Reversal of tubal sterilization. Clin Obstet Gynecol 1980;23:1261.

Wood C, McMaster R, et al: Factors influencing pregnancy rates following in vitro fertilization and embryo transfer. Fertil Steril 1985;43:245.

Woosley RE, Kimg JS, Talbert L: Prolactin-secreting pituitary adenomas: Neurosurgical management of 37 patients. Fertil Steril 1982;37:54.

Yen SSC, Lein A: The apparent paradox of the negative and positive feedback control system on gonadotropin secretion. Am J Obstet Gynecol 1976;126:942.

Zacur HA: Ovulation induction with gonadotropin-releasing hormone. In: Modern Trends in Infertility and Conception Control. Wallach EE, Kempers RD (eds.) Chicago: Year Book Medical Publishers, 1988;4:183-196.

Zamboni L: Sperm ultrastructural pathology and infertility. In: Pathology of Infertility. Gondos B, Riddick D (eds.) New York: Thieme Medical Publishers, 1987;281.